Drug Consultant and Interaction Guide

Mark C. Rathgeber R. Ph., B. Sc. ASCP
Editor
Mark E Schroeder M.D. ACP
Consulting Editor

GW Manning

ATTENTION
The information in this guide is available in computer disk format with printing capabilities. For information contact: Mark Rathgerber, or G.W. Manning & Associates

Disclaimer of warranty: This material is an educational service toward better health care. The creators have attempted to ensure that the drug information and interaction information contained herein accurately reflects published data and is an accordance with standards accepted at the time of publication. Never the less, this is merely a summary of information available from other sources in which specific interactions are analyzed and discussed in more detail. Therefore, the creator of this work shall not be liable for personal injury, property damage, or any consequential damages arising out of or related to the material contained herein. Creators extend no warranties whether expressed or implied as to the completeness of drug information or interactions contained herein.

How to use this guide Simply look up the medication in question in the index by either a trade or generic name. Both names are referenced to a specific chart which describes uses, warnings, side effects, precautions and interaction. When an interaction indicates a change in the effects of a drug, this may also result in a corresponding change in the side effects. In using this reference remember some interacting drugs are used together to treat certain conditions. The serious interactions should be avoided when ever possible unless otherwise directed by physician. The index lists over 2300 drugs by both their trade and (generic) (chemical) name with corresponding charts.

Publisher: Glenn Whaley & Thomas A. Manning
Design Director: Glenn Whaley
Production:
-Layout Design: Angela M. Blackwell
-Cover Design: Glenn Whaley
-Typesetter: Patricia Fitzgerald

Printed in the United States of America

G W Manning
2601 Metro Blvd., St. Louis, MO 63043

Library of Congress Cataloging in Publication Data

Rathgeber, Mark C.
Drug consultant and interaction guide

ISBN 1-876060-04-X

TABLE OF CONTENTS

CHART/TITLES

TABLE OF CONTENTS

CHART 1 : ABUSED & ADDICTIVE COMMON DRUGS

EXAMPLES: Any of these drugs used on any routine basis.
Alcohol - including Wine & Beer.
Nicotine - from smoking; Caffeine - including excess coffee, tea & colas. All are referenced in specific drug charts as are other potentially abused drugs such as; Antianxiety CH.11, Barbiturates CH.23, Stimulants CH.30, Diet Aids CH.33, Narcotic CH.51, & Sedatives CH.59.

INDICATIONS & EFFECTS:
Caffeine - Drowsiness. Nicotine (gum or patch) - Smoking deterrent. The effects of alcohol range from CNS depression to psychological and physical dependence. Nicotine effects are both stimulant and depressant on the CNS, whereas caffeine is a stimulant.

DRUG-DISEASE PRECAUTIONS:
Dependency, Cardiovascular problems, Ulcer, High blood pressure, Diabetes, Kidney or Liver dysfunction. Nicotine (smoking) - Asthma, or breathing difficulties.

DRUG-ALLERGY PRECAUTIONS:
Sensitivity to any ingredients.

PRECAUTIONS:
Routine use may cause addiction, physical problems and with Alcohol - mental health problems, anxiety, confusion, decreased memory including poor judgement and additional health problems.

SIDE EFFECTS: Common with regular use.
REPORT: Irregular heartbeat or blood pressure, persistent diarrhea, confusion, delusions, irrational judgment, stomach pain, anxiety, interrupted sleep patterns, irritability, decreased coordination or libido, mood changes, avoidance, incontinence.
MONITOR: Stomach distress, vision problems, increased or decreased appetite, dizziness or unsteady gait.

***PREGNANCY NURSING AGE STORAGE ABUSE PRECAUTIONS:**
Avoid alcohol and nicotine in pregnancy and nursing. Use moderation with caffeine. Elderly may be more susceptible to effects. All are physically and psychologically addictive with continued use.

Interacting drugs may be used together in some conditions.

DRUG INTERACTIONS FOR: ABUSED AND ADDICTIVE COMMON DRUGS

ALCOHOL PRODUCTS

+ CNS depressants, Anxiety agents, Antihistamines, Barbiturates, Muscle relaxants, Narcotics, Sedatives - **May seriously** increase the side effects of either drug
+ H2 blockers, Cimetidine, Ranitidine - May increase effects of former drug
+ Most all drugs will interact and increase or decrease effects. See specific references in chapters throughout this guide.

CAFFEINE PRODUCTS: Also referenced in CH. 63 and 8, 18,19,21,25,26,30,31,32,33,39,41,45,46,58,60

+ MAO Inhibitors, Theophyllines & Xanthines, Otc Diet Aids, CNS Stimulants, Decongestants - **May seriously** increase effects of latter drug
+ Cimetidine, Ciprofloxacin, Disulfiram, Oral contraceptives - May increase effects of former drug

NICOTINE PRODUCTS (smoking, gums & patches) Also referenced in CH.13,16,34,38,40,51,53,54,63,64,65,67

+ Insulin - **May seriously** increase effects of latter drug
+ Beta Blockers, Bronkodilators, Propoxyphene products - May decrease effects of latter drug (Thus reduction in Nicotine may increase effects of latter drug)

FOOD/NUTRIENT INTERACTIONS:

See specific referenced charts listed above.

RX LABEL PRECAUTIONS:

Alcohol - May cause drowsiness. Avoid in pregnancy.
Caffeine - May cause anxiety. Moderation in pregnancy
Nicotine - Avoid in pregnancy.

***Store all medicines out of childrens reach, away from heat and direct sunlight. Discard old/outdated medications.**
Inform physician(s)/pharmacist of all current medications and any questions that may arise.

See complete prescribing literature for additional information.

CHART 2 : ACE INHIBITORS

EXAMPLES:

ACCUPRIL ALTACE BENAZEPRIL CAPOTEN CAPOZIDE CAPTOPRIL ENALAPRIL FOSINOPRIL LISINOPRIL LOTENSIN MONOPRIL PRINIVIL PRINZIDE QUINAPRIL RAMIPRIL VASERETIC VASOTEC ZESTORETIC ZESTRIL

INDICATIONS & EFFECTS:

Hypertension, Certain heart conditions and other conditions as determined by physician. Effects of Angiotensin 1 converting enzyme inhibitors decrease Angiotensin 2 vasoconstriction effects, increased renin activity with reduction in aldosterone and improved cardiac output.

DRUG-DISEASE PRECAUTIONS:

Angioedema, Lupus, Diabetes, Urinary problems, Hyperkalemia, Low salt diets.

DRUG-ALLERGY PRECAUTIONS:

Sensitivity to any Angiotensin - converting enzyme inhibitors.

PRECAUTIONS:

Potential dizziness, Dehydration, Excess Potassium, (Hyperkalemia, Anxiety, Confusion, Slow Heartbeat, Numbness, Breathing Problems, Weakness), Profuse sweating, Heavy exercise

SIDE EFFECTS: Rare

REPORT: Very low blood pressure, Swelling, Rash, Confusion, Breathing problems, Extreme weakness, Heart problems, Numbness or Tingling

MONITOR: Coughing, Dizziness, Nausea, Headache, Diarrhea, Change in taste

***PREGNANCY/NURSING/AGE/STORAGE/ABUSE PRECAUTIONS:**

Avoid pregnancy or nursing unless otherwise directed. Elderly may be more susceptible to effects.

Interacting drugs may be used together in some conditions.

DRUG INTERACTIONS FOR: ACE INHIBITORS

+ Antacids, Aspirin, Non-Steroidal anti-inflammatory, Decongestants, CNS Stimulants, OTC Diet aids - May decrease effectiveness of former drug
+ Alcohol, Anesthetics inhalation, Diuretics - **May seriously** increase the side effects of either drug
+ Lithium, Insulin, Diabetic agents - **May seriously** increase the side effects of latter drug
+ Potassium products, Potassium sparing diuretics - **May seriously** increase potassium levels and/or side effects of former drug
+ Beta Blockers, other Antihypertensive - May increase effects of either drug.

QUINAPRIL PRODUCTS - In addition

+ Tetracyclines - **May seriously** decrease effectiveness of latter drug

FOOD/NUTRIENT INTERACTIONS:

+ Low salt diets, Salt substitutes, Excess consumption of Potassium products i.e. Bananas, Orange juice - **May seriously** increase potassium level and/or side effects of former drug

RX LABEL PRECAUTIONS:

Take only as directed. DO NOT double dose. Take on empty stomach unless otherwise advised.

***Store all medicines out of childrens reach, away from heat and direct sunlight. Discard old/outdated medications.**
Inform physician(s)/pharmacist of all current medications and any questions that may arise.

See complete prescribing literature for additional information.

CHART 3 : ACETAMINOPHEN ANALGESICS

EXAMPLES:

ACETAMINOPHEN ANACIN-3 APAP DATRIL EXTRA GENEBS LIQUIPRIN PANADOL PHENAPHEN TEMPRA TY-TABS TYLENOL VALADOL

INDICATIONS & EFFECTS:

Analgesics, Pain, Fever and other conditions determined by physician. Effects are through inhibiting prostaglandin synthesis with a resultant decrease in pain and or fever.

DRUG-DISEASE PRECAUTIONS:

Alcoholism, Liver or Urinary problems, Hepatitis

DRUG-ALLERGY PRECAUTIONS:

Sensitivity to Acetaminophen.

PRECAUTIONS:

Avoid alcohol especially if consumed at the same time. May affect blood glucose tests. Do not use other analgesics or pain relievers at the same time unless otherwise directed. Have frequent check ups if using routinely.

SIDE EFFECTS: Rare

REPORT: Severe stomach distress, Pain, Nausea, Swelling and urinary problems

MONITOR: Eye problems, Weakness, Upset stomach

*** PREGNANCY/NURSING/AGE/STORAGE/ABUSE PRECAUTIONS:**

Notify physician if pregnant or nursing. Elderly may be more susceptible to side effects.

Interacting drugs may be used together in some conditions.

DRUG INTERACTIONS FOR: ACETAMINOPHEN ANALGESICS

+ Alcohol, Salicylates, Non steroidal anti-inflammatories - **May seriously** increase side effects of either drug
+ Anticoagulants with high doses of acetaminophen - Possible increase in effects of latter drug
+ Zidovudine - May increase side effects of latter drug

FOOD/NUTRIENT INTERACTIONS:

+ Aspartamine - May increase risks in phenylketonuria patients.

RX LABEL PRECAUTIONS:

Take only as directed. DO NOT double dose. This OTC product IS a drug.

***Store all medicines out of childrens reach, away from heat and direct sunlight. Discard old/outdated medications.**
Inform physician(s)/pharmacist of all current medications and any questions that may arise.

See complete prescribing literature for additional information.

CHART 4 : ADRENERGIC PERIPHERAL ANTIHYPERTENSIVES

EXAMPLES:

DIUPRES ENDURONYL ESIMIL GUANADREL GUANETHIDINE HARMONYL HYDROPRES HYDROSERPINE HYLOREL ISMELIN METATENSIN RAUDIXIN RAUWILOID RAUWOLFIA RAUZIDE REGROTON RESERPINE SALUTENSIN SER-AP-ES SERPASIL

INDICATIONS & EFFECTS:

Hypertension, and some may have other uses as determined by physician. Effects are through decreasing norepinephrine effects and reduced vasoconstriction or cardiac output with a resultant decrease in blood pressure.

DRUG-DISEASE PRECAUTIONS:

Ulcer, colitis, mental depression or other problems, Heart, Urinary, Gallstones

DRUG-ALLERGY PRECAUTIONS:

Sensitivity to any of the ingredients.

PRECAUTIONS:

Rising suddenly from reclined position may cause dizziness.

SIDE EFFECTS: Rare

REPORT: Severe dizziness, Nausea & vomiting, Shortness of breath, Eye problems, Changes in pulse, Unusual bleeding, Swelling

MONITOR: Diarrhea, Mental changes, Weakness, Light headedness, Low blood pressure

* **PREGNANCY/NURSING/AGE/STORAGE/ABUSE PRECAUTIONS:**

Inform physician if pregnant or nursing. Elderly may be more susceptible to side effects. Take only as directed. DO NOT double dose.

Interacting drugs may be used together in some conditions.

DRUG INTERACTIONS FOR: ADRENERGIC PERIPHERAL ANTIHYPERTENSIVES

ALL PRODUCTS

+ Alcohol, Barbiturates, Anxiety & sedative & hypnotic agents - May increase side effects of latter drug
+ Decongestants, CNS stimulants - May decrease effects of former drug
+ Anesthetics - **May seriously** increase the side effects of either drug
+ MAO Inhibitors - **May seriously** increase the side effects of latter drug
+ Antihypertensives - (Other) May increase side effects of either drug
+ Bromocriptine, Levodopa - May decrease effectiveness of latter drug

GUANETHIDINE and GUANADREL - In addition

+ Minoxidil, Diabetic Agents, Insulin - **May seriously** increase side effects of latter drug
+ Antidepressants, Oral contraceptives, Phenothiazines - **May seriously** decrease effects of former drug

FOOD/NUTRIENT INTERACTIONS:

+ Food - May decrease mild nausea if taken with food.

RX LABEL PRECAUTIONS:

Take with food. Avoid alcohol. May cause drowsiness.

***Store all medicines out of childrens reach, away from heat and direct sunlight. Discard old/outdated medications.**
Inform physician(s)/pharmacist of all current medications and any questions that may arise.

See complete prescribing literature for additional information.

CHART 5 : ALKYLATING & ANTIMETABOLITE AGENTS

EXAMPLES:

ADRUCIL ALKERAN BICNU BUSULFAN CARBOPLATIN CARMUSTINE CEENU CHLORAMBUCIL CISPLATIN CYCLOPHOSPHAMIDE CYTOSAR-U CYTOXAN IFEX IFOSFAMIDE FLUDARA FLUOROURACIL FUDR LEUKERAN LOMUSTINE MECHLORETHAMINE MELPHALAM MUSTARGEN MYLERAN NEOSAR NITROGEN MUSTARD PARAPLATIN PIPOBROMAN PLATINOL PURINETHOL STREPTOZOCIN THIOGUANINE THIOTEPA URACIL MUSTARD VERCYTE ZANOSAR

INDICATIONS & EFFECTS:

Hodgkins, Leukemia, Lymphomas, Certain inflammatory conditions and other conditions as determined by physician. Effects are through the disruption of intracellular components, IE: DNA, enzymes and RNA with a resultant decrease in cell proliferation.

DRUG-DISEASE PRECAUTIONS:

Bone Marrow suppression, Renal or Hepatic impairment, Infection, Urinary problems, Chicken pox, Herpes, Gout

DRUG-ALLERGY PRECAUTIONS:

Sensitivity to any alkylating agents.

PRECAUTIONS:

Infections, Joint pain, Vaccines, Must have frequent physician visits to monitor blood and urine tests. Notify any physician seen as to drug and dosage. Take only as directed. Drink plenty of fluids.

SIDE EFFECTS: Moderate

REPORT: Infections, Fever, Heart problems, Bleeding problems or blood in urine, Black stools, Swelling, Jaundice, Confusion

MONITOR: Hair loss, Nausea, Loss of appetite, Diarrhea, Nausea

*** PREGNANCY/NURSING/AGE/STORAGE/ABUSE PRECAUTIONS:**

Avoid pregnancy and nursing. Young and elderly may be more sensitive to side effects.

Interacting drugs may be used together in some conditions.

DRUG INTERACTIONS FOR: ALKYLATING & ANTIMETABOLITE AGENTS
ALL PRODUCTS
+ Antigout agents - **May seriously** decrease effectiveness of latter drug with increased uric acid
+ Cocaine, Other Antineoplastics - **May seriously** increase the side effects of either drug
+ Steroids, Vaccines - May increase risk of infections

CARMUSTINE PRODUCTS - In addition
+ Cimetidine - **May seriously** increase effects of former drug
+ Digoxin, Phenytoin - May decrease effects of latter drug

CISPLATIN PRODUCTS - In addition
+ Aminoglycosides, Loop Diuretics - **May seriously** increase side effects of former drug
+ Phenytoin - May decrease effects of latter drug

CYCLOPHOSPHAMIDE PRODUCTS - In addition
+ Anticoagulants, Doxorubicin, Succinylcholine - **May seriously** increase effects of latter drug
+ Digoxin - May decrease effects of latter drug

CYTARABINE PRODUCTS - In addition
+ Digoxin tabs - May decrease effects of latter drug

FLUOROURACIL PRODUCTS - In addition
+ Cimetidine, Leucovorin - **May seriously** increase effects of former drug

MERCAPTOPURINE PRODUCTS - In addition
+ Allopurinol, SMZ/TMP - **May seriously** increase effects of former drug

FOOD/NUTRIENT INTERACTIONS:
+ Food - Maintain adequate diet, if nauseated eat lighter portions at one time.

FLUOROURACIL (oral)
+ Acidic Juices - May decrease effects of former drug

RX LABEL PRECAUTIONS:

Drink plenty of fluids. Take only as directed. Have frequent check ups.

***Store all medicines out of childrens reach, away from heat and direct sunlight. Inform MD or pharmacist of all current medications.**

See complete prescribing literature for additional information.

CHART 6 : ALPHA-1 PERIPHERAL ANTIHYPERTENSIVES

EXAMPLES:

CARDURA DOXAZOCIN HYTRIN MINIPRESS MINIZIDE PRAZOSIN TERAZOCIN

INDICATIONS & EFFECTS:

Hypertension and other conditions determined by physician. Effects are through vasodilation and improved cardiac output, with a resultant decrease in blood pressure.

DRUG-DISEASE PRECAUTIONS:

Cardiac disease, Urinary problems

DRUG-ALLERGY PRECAUTIONS:

Sensitivity to any ingredients.

PRECAUTIONS:

Avoid alcohol. Irregular heartbeat, Rising from reclined position or extensive exercise may cause dizziness. Do not discontinue without checking with physician. Take first dose at bedtime unless otherwise directed.

SIDE EFFECTS: Rare

REPORT: Chest pain, Shortness of breath, Urinary problems
MONITOR: Weakness, Nausea, Drowsiness

*** PREGNANCY/NURSING/AGE/STORAGE/ABUSE PRECAUTIONS:**

Inform physician if pregnant or nursing. Elderly may be more sensitive to effects of medication.

Interacting drugs may be used together in some conditions.

DRUG INTERACTIONS FOR: ALPHA-1 PERIPHERAL ANTIHYPERTENSIVES

- \+ Alcohol - **May seriously** increase side effects of latter drug
  Antihypertensives, (other) Beta Blockers, Calcium Channel Blockers, Diazoxide - **May seriously** increase the effects of either drug
- \+ Decongestants, CNS Stimulants, OTC Diet aids, Non-steroidal anti-inflammatory agents - May decrease effectiveness of former drug

FOOD/NUTRIENT INTERACTIONS:

Salt - Excessive use may decrease effectiveness of medication

RX LABEL PRECAUTIONS:

Take only as directed. DO NOT double dose. May cause drowsiness.

***Store all medicines out of childrens reach, away from heat and direct sunlight. Discard old/outdated medications.**
Inform physician(s)/pharmacist of all current medications and any questions that may arise.

See complete prescribing literature for additional information.

CHART 7 : ALPHA-2 CENTRAL ANTIHYPERTENSIVES

EXAMPLES:

ALDOCLOR ALDOMET ALDORIL CATAPRES CLONIDINE COMBIPRES GUANABENZ GUANFACINE METHYLDOPA TENEX WYTENSIN

INDICATIONS & EFFECTS:

Hypertension, and other conditions as determined by physician. Effects occur through stimulation of Alpha-2 adrenergic receptors decreasing sympathetic output with resultant blood pressure.

DRUG-DISEASE PRECAUTIONS:

Liver disease, Anemia, Urinary disease, Pheochromocytoma, Heart disease, Depression

DRUG-ALLERGY PRECAUTIONS:

Sensitivity to ingredients, Some Methyldopa products may contain sulfites.

PRECAUTIONS:

Rising suddenly from a reclined position may cause dizziness, Dry mouth, Take only as directed.

SIDE EFFECTS: Rare

REPORT: Swelling, Urinary problems, Severe fever, Nausea and vomiting, Irregular heartbeat.

MONITOR: Weakness, Joint pain, Rash, Headache, Dry mouth, Any change in breathing, drowsiness, decrease libido.

*** PREGNANCY/NURSING/AGE/STORAGE/ABUSE PRECAUTIONS:**

Inform physician if pregnant or nursing. Elderly may be more susceptible to effects.

Interacting drugs may be used together in some conditions.

DRUG INTERACTIONS FOR: ALPHA-2 CENTRAL ANTIHYPERTENSIVES

ALL PRODUCTS

- + Alcohol, Sedatives, Hypnotics, Anxiety Agents, Barbiturates - May increase side effects of either drug
- + Cocaine, Antidepressants, Decongestants, CNS Stimulants, OTC Diet aids - May decrease effectiveness of former drug
- + Antihypertensives - (other) May increase effectiveness of either drug

CLONIDINE PRODUCTS - In addition

- + Beta Blockers - **May seriously** decrease effectiveness of either drug if already on Clonidine, if on both do not discontinue at the same time
- + Levodopa - May decrease effects of latter drug

METHYLDOPA PRODUCTS - In addition

- + MAO Inhibitors, Lithium - **May seriously** increase side effects of latter drug
- + Anticoagulants - May increase effects of latter drug
- + Levodopa - May decrease effects of latter drug
- + Anesthetics - May increase effects of either drug

FOOD/NUTRIENT INTERACTIONS FOR METHYLDOPA:

- + Iron - May decrease effectiveness of former drug if taken at the same time, take 2 hours apart unless otherwise directed.

RX LABEL PRECAUTIONS:

Take only as directed. DO NOT double dose. May cause drowsiness.

***Store all medicines out of childrens reach, away from heat and direct sunlight. Discard old/outdated medications.**

Inform physician(s)/pharmacist of all current medications and any questions that may arise.

See complete prescribing literature for additional information.

CHART 8 : AMINOGLYCOSIDES ORAL/IV

EXAMPLES:

GARAMYCIN GENOPTIC GENTACIDIN GENTAMICIN KANA-MYCIN KANTREX NEOMYCIN

INDICATIONS & EFFECTS:

Antibiotics used in various infections as determined by physician. Effects occur through binding of bacterial ribosomes, with resultant decrease in proliferation of bacterial cell.

DRUG-DISEASE PRECAUTIONS:

Myasthenia gravis, Parkinsonism, Renal problems, Botulism

DRUG-ALLERGY PRECAUTIONS:

Sensitivity to any Aminoglycosides.

PRECAUTIONS:

Serum concentration should be monitored in all patients.

SIDE EFFECTS: Rare to Moderate

REPORT: Any hearing or ear problems, Any Urinary problems, Any dizziness, Nausea/Vomiting, Decreased or difficult breathing.
MONITOR: Minor itching, Minor upset stomach

*** PREGNANCY/NURSING/AGE/STORAGE/ABUSE PRECAUTIONS:**

Avoid pregnancy if at all possible. Notify physician if nursing. Elderly and or young may be much more sensitive to side effects.

Interacting drugs may be used together in some conditions.

DRUG INTERACTIONS FOR: AMINOGLYCOSIDES ORAL/IV

+ Amphotericin B , Loop diuretics, Cephalosporins, Cisplatin, Cyclosporine, Anesthetics, Polymixins, Vancomycin, Magnesium sulfate, Neostigmine, Prostigmine - **May seriously** increase side effects of either drug
+ Narcotics, Malathion - May increase side effects of either drug
+ Methotrexate - **May seriously** increase or decrease the Methotrexate effects
+ Penicillin - May decrease effectiveness of former drug

FOOD/NUTRIENT INTERACTIONS:

+ Dehydration - May increase side effects of former

RX LABEL PRECAUTIONS:

Oral dosage - Take with full glass of water.

***Store all medicines out of childrens reach, away from heat and direct sunlight. Discard old/outdated medications.**
Inform physician(s)/pharmacist of all current medications and any questions that may arise.

See complete prescribing literature for additional information.

CHART 9 : ANABOLIC & ANDROGENIC STEROIDS

EXAMPLES:

ANADROL ANDROID DANAZOL DANOCRINE FLUOXY-MESTERONE HALOTESTIN METANDREN METHYLTEST-OSTER OXYMETHOLONE STANOZOLOL TESTRED WINSTROL

INDICATIONS & EFFECTS:

Antianemic, Antineoplastic, Angioedema and other conditions as determined by physician. Use in athletic or weight endeavors is NOT an indication and should be avoided since there are serious side effects. Effects occur through replacing natural anabolic or androgenic steroids and metabolism.

DRUG-DISEASE PRECAUTIONS:

Diabetes, Breast cancer, Heart problems, Liver problems, Prostate problems

DRUG-ALLERGY PRECAUTIONS:

Sensitivity to any of the ingredients.

PRECAUTIONS:

Decrease in Blood sugar, Fertility may be decreased. Must have regular check ups.

SIDE EFFECTS: Moderate

REPORT: Menstrual problems, Edema, Unusual bleeding, Nausea, Vomiting, Liver, Urinary, Eye problems, Headache, Dizziness, Shortness of breath, Rash, Severe itching, Depression, Tiredness

MONITOR: Stomach upset, Restlessness, Impotence, Change in Libido, Diarrhea, Constipation, Sun sensitivity

*** PREGNANCY/NURSING/AGE/STORAGE/ABUSE PRECAUTIONS:**

DO NOT use if pregnant or nursing unless otherwise directed. Elderly may be more susceptible to effects. Use in pre-adults not recommended due to change in bone growth.

Interacting drugs may be used together in some conditions.

DRUG INTERACTIONS FOR: ANABOLIC & ANDROGENIC STEROIDS
+ Other Steroids - May increase side effects of either drug
+ Anticoagulants, Cyclosporine - May increase the side effects of latter drug
+ Diabetic Agents, Insulin - **May seriously** increase effects of latter drug

FOOD/NUTRIENT INTERACTIONS:
+ Excess salt and Excessive sodium Containing Products such as Bacon, Ham, Soups, Bouillon, Pickles, Snack foods, Sardines, Some canned vegetables and frozen foods - May cause excess fluid retention

RX LABEL PRECAUTIONS:

Take with food. Take only as directed. DO NOT double dose. Use Sun screen when outside for prolong periods.

***Store all medicines out of childrens reach, away from heat and direct sunlight. Discard old/outdated medications.**
Inform physician(s)/pharmacist of all current medications and any questions that may arise.

See complete prescribing literature for additional information.

CHART 10 : ANTACIDS

EXAMPLES:

BASALJEL BISMUTH SUBSALICYLATE CALCIUM CARBONATE DI-GEL GAVISCON GELUSIL MAALOX MAGALDRATE MYLANTA PEPTO-BISMOL RIOPAN ROLAIDS SF TITRALAC TUMS

INDICATIONS & EFFECTS:

Antacid, Laxative, Ulcer, Reflux, Hypocalcium, and other conditions as determined by physician. Effects occur through decreasing or neutralizing stomach acidity, magnesium containing products may cause laxative effect and aluminum or calcium products may cause a constipation.

DRUG-DISEASE PRECAUTIONS:

Hypercalcemia, Urinary problems, Appendicitis, Liver problems, Chronic diarrhea

DRUG-ALLERGY PRECAUTIONS:

Sensitivity to any ingredients.

PRECAUTIONS:

Possible constipation with Aluminum or Calcium containing products. Diarrhea with Magnesium containing products. Take 1 to 2 hours after or before other medications unless otherwise directed. Constipation/Diarrhea, Sodium content with low salt diet.

SIDE EFFECTS: Rare

REPORT: Extreme tiredness, Dizziness, Mental changes, Urinary problems, Cardiac changes, Nausea and Vomiting, Breathing problems

MONITOR: Mild Constipation or Diarrhea, Cramps, Increased thirst

* **PREGNANCY/NURSING/AGE/STORAGE/ABUSE PRECAUTIONS**:

Inform physician if pregnant/nursing. Elderly may be more susceptible to effects.

Interacting drugs may be used together in some conditions.

DRUG INTERACTIONS FOR: ANTACIDS

NOTE: Take Antacid 1 to 2 hours after other drugs unless otherwise directed.

+ Tetracyclines, Anxiety Agents, Antiulcer Agents, Ace Inhibitors, Steroids, Digitalis, Fluroquinolones, Ketoconazole, Metronidazole, Nitrofurantoin, Penicillamines, Digestants with Calcium or Magnesium Antacids, Anticholinergies - **May seriously** decrease effects of latter drug if taken at the same time, take 2 hours after, unless otherwise directed
+ Quinine, Quinidine, Theophyllines, Xanthines - **May seriously** increase effects of latter drug with large doses of Antacids
+ Allopurinol, Phenytoin, Isoniazid, Fluoride, Beta Blockers, Salicylates - May decrease effectiveness of latter drug with Calcium or Aluminum Antacids taken at the same time, take 2 hours apart

BISMUTH SUBSALICYLATE PRODUCTS - In addition

+ Methotrexate - **May seriously** increase effects of latter drug, avoid using Subsalicylate products.

FOOD/NUTRIENT INTERACTIONS:

+ Iron - May decrease effects of latter if taken at the same time
+ Low salt diet - May decrease effects of low salt diet if antacid is high in Sodium content

NOTE: Certain amounts of the specific ingredients i.e. Aluminum, Calcium or Magnesium may be absorbed when taking antacids

RX LABEL PRECAUTIONS:

DO NOT take with other medications unless otherwise directed. Take 1 to 2 hours after. Shake liquids well.

***Store all medicines out of childrens reach, away from heat and direct sunlight. Discard old/outdated medications.**
Inform physician(s)/pharmacist of all current medications and any questions that may arise.

See complete prescribing literature for additional information.

CHART 11 : ANTIANXIETY AND SEDATIVE AGENTS

EXAMPLES:

ALPRAZOLAM ATIVAN BUSPAR CENTRAX CHLORDIAZEPOXIDE CLORAZEPATE DALMANE DIAZEPAM ESTAZOLAM FLURAZEPAM HALAZEPAM HALCION KLONOPIN LIBRITABS LIBRIUM LORAZEPAM OXAZEPAM PAXIPAM PRAZEPAM PROSOM RESTORIL SERAX TEMAZEPAM TRANXENE TRIAZOLAM VALIUM VALRELEASE XANAX

INDICATIONS & EFFECTS:

Anxiety, Sedative, Hypnotic, Skeletal muscle relaxant, Anticonvulsant, Antinausea, and other conditions. Effects occur through CNS depression muscle relaxation and may result in dependency with continued use.

DRUG-DISEASE PRECAUTIONS:

Alcoholism, Kidney or Liver problems, Glaucoma, Mental depression, Myasthenia gravis, Breathing problems. Drug dependency history or abuse.

DRUG-ALLERGY PRECAUTIONS:

Sensitivity to any ingredients.

PRECAUTIONS:

Alcohol and any other CNS depressants, Drug dependency history or abuse, Decreased respiration, Drowsiness, Unsteadiness, Possible withdrawal (Nervousness, Mental changes, Fast heartbeat, Confusion, Sleeplessness) - Dosage should be decreased gradually over a 2-6 week period. Buspirone may be less likely to cause these effects.

SIDE EFFECTS: Moderate

REPORT: Confusion, Irregular heartbeat, Severe drowsiness or weakness, Irritability, Restlessness, Nausea or vomiting

MONITOR: Mild drowsiness, Lightheadedness, Upset stomach, unusual tiredness

*** PREGNANCY/NURSING/AGE/STORAGE/ABUSE PRECAUTIONS:**

Inform physician if pregnant or nursing. Best avoided if pregnant unless otherwise directed by physician. Elderly and children may be more sensitive to effects. May be habit forming. Avoid long term use unless otherwise directed.

Interacting drugs may be used together in some conditions.

DRUG INTERACTIONS FOR: ANTIANXIETY AND SEDATIVE AGENTS
ALL PRODUCTS

+ Alcohol, Barbiturates, Fluoxetine, Hypnotics, Narcotics, Sedatives, Tricyclic Antidepressants - **May seriously** increase side effects of either drug

BENZODIAZEPINE PRODUCTS - In addition

+ Cimetidine, Disulfiram, Omeprazole, Probenecid, Ranitidine - **May seriously** increase effects of former drug
+ Erythromycin, Ketoconazole, Beta Blockers - May increase effects of former drug
+ Levodopa products - May decrease effects of latter drug
+ Amiodarone, Loxapine - May increase effects of latter drug

BUSPRIONE PRODUCTS - In addition

+ Digoxin, Fluoxetine - May increase effects of latter drug
+ MAO Inhibitors - **May seriously** increase effects of latter drug (Allow 2 weeks between MAO therapy before Busprione)

FOOD/NUTRIENT INTERACTIONS:

+ Food - Less stomach upset if taken with food

RX LABEL PRECAUTIONS:

May cause drowsiness - Use caution driving and operating machinery. Avoid alcohol. DO NOT double dose.

***Store all medicines out of childrens reach, away from heat and direct sunlight. Discard old/outdated medications.**
Inform physician(s)/pharmacist of all current medications and any questions that may arise.

See complete prescribing literature for additional information.

CHART 12 : ANTICHOLINERGICS & ANTISPASMODICS

EXAMPLES:

ANASPAZ BELLADONNA BENTYL BUTIBEL CLINDEX CYSTOSPAZ DICYCLOMINE DONNATAL LEVSIN LIBRAX PAMINE PATHILON PRO-BANTHINE PROPANTHELINE QUARZAN ROBINUL

INDICATIONS & EFFECTS:

Ulcer, Urinary problems, Motion sickness, Intestinal problems, Allergies, Antispasmodic, Certain cardiac conditions and other conditions as determined by physician. Effects occur through decreased nerve stimulation.

DRUG-DISEASE PRECAUTIONS:

Down's Syndrome, Fever, Glaucoma, Bleeding problems, Urinary or Liver problems, Myasthenia gravis, Hernia, Heart problems.

DRUG-ALLERGY PRECAUTIONS:

Sensitivity to any ingredients.

PRECAUTIONS:

Monitor: Intraocular pressure may increase in patients over 40 - Pupil dilation with scopolamine. All products may increase body temperature, Use caution when exercising, Dizziness, Drowsiness.

SIDE EFFECTS: Moderate

REPORT: Vision problems, Confusion, Low blood pressure, Extreme dizziness, Tiredness, Change in heart rate, Shortness of breath

MONITOR: Constipation, Dry mouth, Headache, Urinary problems, Nausea or Vomiting, Weakness or Drowsiness

* **PREGNANCY/NURSING/AGE/STORAGE/ABUSE PRECAUTIONS:**

Best Avoided if Pregnant or nursing, unless otherwise directed. May decrease lactation. Infants and young are more susceptible to side effects - Best avoided. May increase Body temperature. Geriatrics more susceptible and in addition may cause agitation or memory problems.

Interacting drugs may be used together in some conditions.

DRUG INTERACTIONS FOR: ANTICHOLINERGICS & ANTISPASMODICS
ALL PRODUCTS

+ Alcohol, Amantadine, Antidepressants, - May cause confusion, nightmares
+ MAO Inhibitors, Carbonic Anhydrase Inhibitors, Urinary Alkalizers - May increase effects of former drug
+ Phenothiazines, Levodopa, Haloperidol, Cimetidine - May decrease effects of latter drug
+ Reserpine, Guanadrel, Guanethidine, Antacids - May decrease effects of former drug
+ Ranitidine, Potassium tabs - May increase side effects of latter drug

SCOPOLAMINE PRODUCTS - In addition

+ Sedatives, Anxiety Agents, Hypnotics, Narcotics - May increase side effects of latter drug

FOOD/NUTRIENT INTERACTIONS:

+ Food - May decrease effects of former drug. Take dosage 1/2 hour before eating unless otherwise directed.

RX LABEL PRECAUTIONS:

Take only as directed. May cause drowsiness. Alcohol may intensify this effect. DO NOT double dose.

***Store all medicines out of childrens reach, away from heat and direct sunlight. Discard old/outdated medications.**
Inform physician(s)/pharmacist of all current medications and any questions that may arise.

See complete prescribing literature for additional information.

CHART 13 : ANTICOAGULANTS

EXAMPLES:

COUMADIN DICUMAROL PANWARFIN SOFARIN WARFARIN

INDICATIONS & EFFECTS:

Circulatory coagulation problems, Myocardial Infarction and other conditions determined by physician. Effects occur through decreased pro-factors mediated by vitamin K.

DRUG-DISEASE PRECAUTIONS:

Clotting deficiencies, Diabetes, Urinary or Liver problems, Vitamin C or K Deficient, Surgery, Abortion, Edema, Ulceration

DRUG-ALLERGY PRECAUTIONS:

Sensitivity to any ingredients.

PRECAUTIONS:

Inform all your physicians or pharmacists you are taking this medication and any over the counter drugs you take. Have frequent check ups, and pro time checks. Exercise caution not to be injured. Maintain a balanced diet.

SIDE EFFECTS: Rare to Moderate

REPORT: Unusual bleeding, Blood in Urine or Stools, Severe Headaches, Swelling, Cramps, Fever, Extreme weakness, Sores, Nausea or Vomiting

MONITOR: Loss of appetite, Gas

*** PREGNANCY/NURSING/AGE/STORAGE/ABUSE PRECAUTIONS:**

Best avoided if pregnant or nursing unless otherwise directed. Elderly may be more susceptible to side effects.

Interacting drugs may be used together in some conditions.

DRUG INTERACTIONS FOR: ANTICOAGULANTS

+ Acetaminophen, Allopurinol, Anabolic and Androgenic Steroids, H2 Blockers, Chloramphenicol, Cimetidine, Clofibrate, Chloral Hydrate, Disulfiram, Erythomycins, Fluroquinolones, Antidiabetic Agents, Ketoconzole, Metronidazole, Methotrexate, Phenylbutazone, Quinine, Quinidine, Sulfas, Sulfinpyrazone, Tamoxifen, Tetracyclines, Thyroids, Triclofos - **May seriously** increase the effects of former drug
+ Barbiturates, Carbamazepine, Cholestyramine, Glutethimide, Griseofulvin, Oral Contraceptives, Penicillin, Rifampin, Spironolactone, Sucralfate, Smoking - **May seriously** decrease the effects of former drug
+ Alcohol, Phenytoin - **May seriously** increase or decrease the effects of former drug
+ Aspirin, Non Steroidal Anti inflammatory Agents, Salicylates - **May seriously** increase the side effects of either drug & potential bleeding

FOOD/NUTRIENT INTERACTIONS:

+ Vitamin K and foods high in Vitamin K in large consumption i.e. Leafy green vegetables, Vitamin C - May decrease effects of former
+ Vitamin A, Vitamin E in large doses - May increase effects of former

RX LABEL PRECAUTIONS:

Avoid alcohol. Take only as directed. DO NOT double dose.

***Store all medicines out of childrens reach, away from heat and direct sunlight. Discard old/outdated medications.**
Inform physician(s)/pharmacist of all current medications and any questions that may arise.
See complete prescribing literature for additional information.

CHART 14 : ANTICONVULSANTS 1

EXAMPLES:

DEPAKENE DEPAKOTE DILANTIN DIVALPROEX ETHOTOIN MEPHENYTOIN MESANTOIN PEGANONE PHENYTOIN VALPROIC ACID

INDICATIONS & EFFECTS:

Convulsion, Muscular disorders and other conditions as determined by physician. Effects occur through stabilizing nerve impulses.

DRUG-DISEASE PRECAUTIONS:

Liver or renal problems, Blood dyscrasias
Hydantoins in addition - Cardiac problems, Diabetes
Valproic Acid + Divalproex in addition - Bleeding disorders

DRUG-ALLERGY PRECAUTIONS:

Sensitivity to any ingredients

PRECAUTIONS:

May cause drowsiness, Alcohol should be avoided, Proper dental hygiene, Do Not double dose, Take only as directed, Have frequent check ups

SIDE EFFECTS: Rare

REPORT: Vision problems, Increased seizures, Mood changes, Persistent nausea or vomiting, Unusual bleeding, Severe cramps, Confusion, Trembling, Severe rash, Sore throat, Weakness, Dark urine, Jaundice, Dizziness, Swelling, Urinary problems

MONITOR: Loss of appetite, Cramps, Diarrhea, Indigestion, Drowsiness, Constipation, Restlessness, Hiccups, Dry mouth

*** PREGNANCY/NURSING/AGE/STORAGE/ABUSE PRECAUTIONS:**

Inform physician immediately if pregnant. Children and elderly may be more sensitive to effects.

***Store all medicines out of childrens reach, away from heat and direct sunlight. Discard old/outdated medications.**
Inform physician(s)/pharmacist of all current medications and any questions that may arise.

See complete prescribing literature for additional information.

Interacting drugs may be used together in some conditions.

DRUG INTERACTIONS FOR: ANTICONVULSANTS 1

ALL PRODUCTS

+ Alcohol, Antianxiety Agents, Barbiturates, Narcotics - **May seriously** increase side effects of latter drug
+ Antacids - May decrease effectiveness of former drug, Take 2 hours apart

HYDANTOINS PRODUCTS - In addition

+ Estrogens-Contraceptives, Levodopa, Methadone, Steroids, Streptozocin, Valproic Acid - **May seriously** decrease effects of latter drug
+ Diazoxide, Theophyllines, Xanthines - **May seriously** decrease effects of either drug
+ Amiodrone, Anticoagulants, Chloramphenicol, Cimetidine, Disulfiram, Isoniazid, Phenylbutazone, Ranitidine, Sulfas, Valproic Acid - **May seriously** increase effects of former drug
+ Alcohol, Antianxiety Agents, Lithium - **May seriously** increase effects of latter drug
+ Ketoconazole, Metronidazole, Omeprazole - May increase effects of latter drug
+ Carbamazepine, Diabetic Agents, Digitalis, Disopyramide, Furosemide, Insulin, Methadone, Mexiletine, Quinidine, Succinimides - May decrease effects of latter drug
+ Antidepressants, Folic Acid, Leucovorin, MAO Inhibitors, Rifampin, Sucralfate, Tranquilizers - May decrease effectiveness of former drug

DIVALPROEX + VALPROIC ACID PRODUCTS- In addition

+ Anti-Inflammatory Agents, Salicylates - **May seriously** increase side effects of latter drug
+ Cimetidine - **May seriously** increase effects of former drug
+ Carbamazepine, Mefloquine - **May seriously** decrease effectiveness of former drug
+ Ethosuximide, Isoniazid, Phenytoin, Primidone - May increase effects of latter drug

FOOD/NUTRIENT INTERACTIONS: HYDANTOINS

+ Calcium Supplements, Excess caffeine, Folic Acid - May decrease effects of former drug
+ Vitamin D - May decrease effects of latter nutrient

RX LABEL PRECAUTIONS:

May cause drowsiness, Avoid alcohol, May take with food if upsetting to stomach.

CHART 15 : ANTICONVULSANTS 2

EXAMPLES:

CARBAMAZEPINE CELONTIN ETHOSUXIMIDE MILONTIN MYSOLINE PRIMIDONE TEGRETOL TRIDIONE TRIMETHADIONE ZARONTIN

INDICATIONS & EFFECTS:

Convulsion, Muscular disorders and other conditions as determined by physician. Effects occur through stabilizing nerve impulses.

DRUG-DISEASE PRECAUTIONS:

Liver or renal problems, Blood dyscrasias. Carbamazepine in addition: Cardiac problems, Diabetes, Glaucoma. Primidones in addition: Respiratory problems

DRUG-ALLERGY PRECAUTIONS:

Sensitivity to any ingredients. Carbamazepine in addition: Sensitivity to Tricyclic Antidepressants. Primidone in addition: Sensitivity to Barbiturates

PRECAUTIONS:

May cause drowsiness, Avoid Alcohol, Proper dental hygiene, Do Not double dose, Take only as directed, Have frequent check ups

SIDE EFFECTS: Rare to Moderate

REPORT: Vision problems, Increased seizures, Mood changes, Persistent nausea or vomiting, Unusual bleeding, Severe cramps, Confusion, Trembling, Severe rash, Sore throat, Weakness, Dark urine, Jaundice, Dizziness, Swelling, Urinary or Breathing problems

MONITOR: Loss of appetite, Cramps, Diarrhea, Indigestion, Drowsiness, Constipation, Restlessness, Hiccups, Dry mouth

*** PREGNANCY/NURSING/AGE/STORAGE/ABUSE PRECAUTIONS:**

Inform physician immediately if pregnant. Children and elderly may be more sensitive to effects.

***Store all medicines out of childrens reach, away from heat and direct sunlight. Inform physician(s) or pharmacist of all current medications and any questions that may arise.**

See complete prescribing literature for additional information.

Interacting drugs may be used together in some conditions.

DRUG INTERACTIONS FOR: ANTICONVULSANTS 2

ALL PRODUCTS

+ Alcohol, Antianxiety Agents, Barbiturates, Narcotics - **May seriously** increase side effects of latter drug
+ Antacids - May decrease effectiveness of former drug, Take two hours apart

SUCCINIMIDES PRODUCTS - In addition

+ Haloperidol - **May seriously** decrease effectiveness of former drug
+ Antidepressants, MAO Inhibitors, Tranquilizers - May decrease effects of former drug
+ Carbamazepine, Divalproex, Phenobarbital, Phenytoin, Prini-done, Valproic Acid - May decrease effectiveness of former drug

DIONES PRODUCTS- - In addition

+ Acetazolamide - May increase side effects of either drug
+ Antidepressants, MAO Inhibitors, Tranquilizers - May decrease effects of former drug

CARBAMAZEPINES PRODUCTS - In addition

+ Anticoagulants, Barbiturates, Estrogens-Contraceptives, Hydantoins, Mexiletine, Primidone, Quinidine, Succinimides, Valproates - **May seriously** decrease effects of latter drug
+ Antidepressants, Cimetidine, Dittiazem, Doxycycline, Erythromycin, Flu vaccine, Isoniazid, Propoxyphene, Troleandomycin, Verapamil - **May seriously** increase effects of former drug

PRIMIDONES PRODUCTS - In addition

+ Anticoagulants, Estrogens-Contraceptives, Mexilitene, Quinidine, Steroids - **May seriously** decrease effects of latter drug
+ MAO Inhibitors, Methylphenidate - **May seriously** increase effects of former drug
+ Carbamazepine **- May seriously** decrease effects of former drug
+ Alcohol, Carbonic Anhydrase Inhibitors, Ethacrynic Acid, Guanadrel, Guanethidine, Phenobarbital - May increase effects of latter drug
+ Caffeine, Theophylline, Xanthines - May decrease effectiveness of latter drug

FOOD/NUTRIENT INTERACTIONS:

CARBAMAZEPINE, DIONES, SUCCINIMIDES PRODUCTS -

+ Folic Acid - May decrease effects of latter nutrient

PRIMIDONES PRODUCTS -

+ Vitamin C (Ascorbic Acid), Vitamin B12, Vitamin D - May decrease effects of latter nutrient

RX LABEL PRECAUTIONS: May cause drowsiness, Avoid alcohol.

CHART 16 : ANTIDEPRESSANTS

EXAMPLES:

AMITRIPTYLINE AMOXAPINE ANAFRANIL ASENDIN AVENTYL BUPROPION CLOMIPRAMINE DESIPRAMINE DESYREL DOXEPIN ELAVIL ENDEP ETRAFON FLUOXETINE IMIPRAMINE LUDIOMIL MAPROTILINE NORPRAMIN NORTRIPTYLINE PAMELOR PROZAC SINEQUAN SERTRALINE SURMONTIL TOFRANIL TRAZODONE TRIAVIL TRIMIPRAMINE VIVACTIL WELLBUTRIN ZOLOFT

INDICATIONS & EFFECTS:

Anxiety, Depression and other conditions as determined by physician. Effects occur through increased levels of norepinephrine or serotonin by blocking reuptake.

DRUG-DISEASE PRECAUTIONS:

Myocardial infarction recovery, Glaucoma or urinary retention with Doxepin products, Seizure disorders with Maprotiline

DRUG-ALLERGY PRECAUTIONS:

Sensitivity to any ingredients

PRECAUTIONS:

Avoid Alcohol, Tardive dyskinesia, Involuntary movements, Cardiovascular disease, Sun sensitivity - Use sunscreen

SIDE EFFECTS: Rare to Moderate

REPORT: Bladder problems, Changes in blood pressure, Difficult breathing, Fever, Muscle stiffness, Numbness or tingling, Priapism

MONITOR: Drowsiness, Vision problems, Confusion, Agitation, Dry mouth, Dizziness, Insomnia, Skin Rash, Nausea, Sexual dysfunction

* **PREGNANCY/NURSING/AGE/STORAGE/ABUSE PRECAUTIONS**:

Notify physician if pregnant or nursing - may need to avoid, Elderly may be more susceptible to effects, Most not used in children less than 18 years of age. Unless otherwise directed by physician.

Interacting drugs may be used together in some conditions.

DRUG INTERACTIONS FOR: ANTIDEPRESSANTS

ALL PRODUCTS

+ MAO Inhibitors - **May seriously** increase effects of latter drug. Avoid concurrent use.
+ Alcohol, Antidepressants, Anticholinergics, Antianxiety Agents, Barbiturates, Tranquilizers - **May seriously** increase effects of latter drug

BUPROPION PRODUCTS - In addition

+ Carbamazepine, Cimetidine, Phenytoin - May decrease effects of latter drug
+ Levodopa - May increase effects of former drug

FLUOXETINE PRODUCTS - In addition

+ Antidepressants, Antidiabetics, Digitoxin, Lithium, L-Tryptophan, Warfarin - **May seriously** increase effects of latter drug

TRAZODONE PRODUCTS - In addition

+ Digoxin, Phenytoin - May increase effects of latter drug

ALL OTHER PRODUCTS - In addition

+ Alcohol, Clonidine, Guanethidine, Dicumarol, Disulfiram - **May seriously** increase effects of either. Avoid concurrent use.
+ Cimetidine, Oral contraceptives, Haloperidol - May increase effects of former drug
+ Levodopa - May decrease effects of latter drug
+ Smoking - May decrease effectiveness of former drug

FOOD/NUTRIENT INTERACTIONS:

FLUOXETINE PRODUCTS

+ L-Tryptophan - **May seriously** increase effects of former drug

RX LABEL PRECAUTIONS:

May cause drowsiness, Avoid alcohol, Use sunscreen when outside for prolonged periods. Take Fluoxetine in AM unless otherwise directed to reduce sleeplessness

***Store all medicines out of childrens reach, away from heat and direct sunlight. Discard old/outdated medications. Inform physician(s) or pharmacist of all current medications and any questions that may arise.**

See complete prescribing literature for additional information.

CHART 17 : ANTIHISTAMINES

EXAMPLES:

ACTIDIL ASTEMIZOLE ATARAX BENADRYL BENYLIN BROMPHENIRAMINE CHLORPHENIRAMINE CHLOR-TRIMETON CLISTIN CYPROHEPTADINE DIMETANE DIPHEN-HYDRAMINE DRAMAMINE HISMANAL HYDRAMINE HYDROXYZINE NOLAHIST OPTIMINE PBZ PERIACTIN PHENERGAN POLARAMINE SELDANE TAVIST TERFENADINE UNISOM VISTARIL

INDICATIONS & EFFECTS:

Allergies, Allergic reactions, Sneezing, Runny nose, Anxiety, Parkinsonism, Cough, Motion sickness, Nausea & Vomiting, Insomnia, and other conditions determined by physician. Effects occur through blocking the action of histamine and some on serotonin this decreasing secreations.

DRUG-DISEASE PRECAUTIONS:

Glaucoma, Urinary retention/obstruction, Acute asthma, Prostatic conditions, Liver problems

DRUG-ALLERGY PRECAUTIONS:

Sensitivity to any Antihistamine

PRECAUTIONS:

Increased sun sensitivity, May cause severe drowsiness especially with other CNS depressant drugs, Do Not double dose.

SIDE EFFECTS: Moderate

REPORT: Irregular heart beat, Unusual bleeding, Sore throat & fever, Severe drowsiness or disorientation, Shortness of breath.
MONITOR: Drowsiness, Rash, Ringing in ears, Eye problems or dryness, Confusion, Agitation or restlessness, More likely in young.

*** PREGNANCY/NURSING/AGE/STORAGE/ABUSE PRECAUTIONS:**

Inform physician if pregnant, may need to avoid nursing, because of effects on child. Some antihistamines may decrease lactation. Elderly may be more sensitive to effects. **Keep out of reach of children.**

Interacting drugs may be used together in some conditions.

DRUG INTERACTIONS FOR: ANTIHISTAMINES
ALL PRODUCTS

Note: Astemizole, Hismanal, Terfenadine, Seldane - **NEVER** take more than prescribed and they may be less likely to produce some of these effects, and drowsiness.

+ Alcohol, Antidepressants, Barbiturates, Benzodiazepines, Anticonvulsants, Narcotics, Muscle relaxants, Antihypertensives, Sedatives, Antianxiety drugs - **May seriously** increase the side effects of either drug
+ Anticholinergics - **May seriously** increase the effects of latter drug
+ MAO Inhibitors - **May seriously** increase the effects of former drug
+ Calcium Blockers - May increase effects of latter drug

TERFENADINE PRODUCTS - In addition

+ Ketoconazole, Troleandomycin, Erythromycin - **May seriously** increase side effects of former drug

FOOD/NUTRIENT INTERACTIONS:

+ Food with Hismanal, Astemizole, - may decrease absorption of antihistamine, and thus effectiveness. Others may be taken with food if they tend to upset stomach.

RX LABEL PRECAUTIONS:

May cause drowsiness - Use caution driving & operating machinery.
NEVER Double Dose.

***Store all medicines out of childrens reach, away from heat and direct sunlight. Discard old/outdated medications.**
Inform physician(s)/pharmacist of all current medications and any questions that may arise.

See complete prescribing literature for additional information.

CHART 18 : ANTIHISTAMINE & DECONGESTANT COMBINATIONS

EXAMPLES:

A.R.M. ACTIFED ALLEREST ALLERFRIN CONTAC DECONAMINE DIMETAPP DISOBROM DISOPHROL DRISTAN DRIXORAL EXTENDRYL ISOCLOR NALDECON NOLAMINE NOVAFED A NOVAHISTINE ORNADE PHENERGAN VC POLY-HISTINE-D RESAID S.R. RONDEC RYNATAN SELDANE-D SINGLET SINUTAB SUDAFED PLUS TAVIST-D TRIAMINIC TRINALIN

INDICATIONS & EFFECTS:

Allergies, Allergic reactions, Sneezing, Sinus headache, Nasal congestion, Cough, Nausea, Runny nose, and other conditions determined by physician. Effects occur by blocking histamine, (reduced secretions), and reducing swelling through vasoconstriction.

DRUG-DISEASE PRECAUTIONS:

Acute Asthma, Urinary problems, Prostatic conditions, Heart problems, Diabetes, Hypertension, Hyperthyroidism, Glaucoma

DRUG-ALLERGY PRECAUTIONS:

Sensitivity to Antihistamines (See chart 17), Decongestants (See chart 33), and CNS stimulants ie: adrenalin, amphetamines, terbutaline

PRECAUTIONS:

May increase sun sensitivity, may cause drowsiness especially if taking other CNS depressants, Possible restlessness, especially if taking other CNS stimulants such as appetite suppressants and caffeine

SIDE EFFECTS: Moderate

REPORT: Increase in blood pressure, Sore throat, Severe headache, Shortness of breath, Severe nausea, Drowsiness, or Confusion and mood changes

MONITOR: Fever, Ear or vision problems, Difficulty sleeping, Tiredness

*** PREGNANCY/NURSING/AGE/STORAGE/ABUSE PRECAUTIONS:**

Inform physician if pregnant, May need to avoid nursing because of effects on child, some antihistamines can decrease lactation. Possible increased reactions in elderly, Possible agitation in young, overdose is dangerous.

Interacting drugs may be used together in some conditions.

DRUG INTERACTIONS FOR: ANTIHISTAMINE & DECONGESTANT
(See also Antihistamines Ch. 17 and Decongestants Ch. 33)

+ Alcohol, Antidepressants, CNS Depressants, Barbiturates, Antianxiety drugs, Cough and cold remedies, Narcotics, Muscle relaxants - May cause increase in side effects of either drug
+ Digoxin, Anesthetics - May increase side effects of former drug
+ Anticholinergics - **May seriously** increase side effects of latter drug
+ Beta Blockers, Guanadrel, Guanethidine - **May seriously** decrease the effectiveness of latter drug
+ Brochodilators, Cocaine, MAO Inhibitors, Theophyllines - **May seriously** increase the side effects of either drug
+ Insulin - May decrease effects of latter drug

FOOD/NUTRIENT INTERACTIONS:

+ Large consumption of coffee, soda and tea - May increase effects of either

RX LABEL PRECAUTIONS:

May cause drowsiness. Take only as directed - DO NOT double dose. Use caution driving and operating machinery.

***Store all medicines out of childrens reach, away from heat and direct sunlight. Discard old/outdated medications.**
Inform physician(s)/pharmacist of all current medications and any questions that may arise.

See complete prescribing literature for additional information.

CHART 19 : ANTIPARKINSON AGENTS

EXAMPLES:

AMANTADINE DOPAR ELDEPRYL LARODOPA LEVODOPA LEVODOPA + CARBIDOPA PERGOLIDE PERMAX SELEGILINE SINEMET SYMMETREL

INDICATIONS & EFFECTS:

Parkinsonism and other conditions as determined by physician ie: Amatadine - May be indicated in flu conditions. Effects are through stimulation or replacing dopamine in the brain; and for Eldepryl, Selegiline - MAO B inhibition.

DRUG-DISEASE PRECAUTIONS:

Asthma, Glaucoma, Heart, Melanoma, Psychotic conditions, Ulcer, Urinary problems; Amatadine - additionally Edema or Epilepsy

DRUG-ALLERGY PRECAUTIONS:

Sensitivity to ingredients & Ergot Alkaloids with Permax (Pergolide)

PRECAUTIONS:

Dizziness, Excessive hypertension and dry mouth with Eldepryl (see MAO Inhibitor chart when Eldepryl is used in high doses). Elderly should exercise caution when returning to more normal activities. Avoid alcohol especially with Symmetrel/Amatadine.

SIDE EFFECTS: Moderate

Report: Hypertension, Uncontrolled movements, Mood changes, Irregular heart beat, Difficult urination, Eye problems, Nausea or vomiting, Stiff neck, Chest pain.

Monitor: weakness anxiety sleeplessness dry mouth diarrhea constipation. May decrease saliva. Anticholinergic effects with Symmetrel/Amatadine

*** PREGNANCY/NURSING/AGE/STORAGE/ABUSE PRECAUTIONS:**

Inform physician if pregnant/nursing. Drugs may inhibit lactation. Elderly may require lower dosages.

***Store all medicines out of childrens reach, away from heat and direct sunlight. Discard old/outdated medications. Inform physician(s) or pharmacist of all current medications and any questions that may arise.**

See complete prescribing literature for additional information.

Interacting drugs may be used together in some conditions.

DRUG INTERACTIONS FOR: ANTIPARKINSON AGENTS

LEVODOPA PRODUCTS:

+ Cocaine - **May Seriously** Increaserisk of arrhythmias
+ Benzodiazepines, Papaverine, Phenothiazines - **May Seriously** decrease in former drugs effectiveness
+ Anticholinergics, Antidepressants, Clonidine, Methyldopa, Phenytoin - Decrease in former drugs effectiveness
+ MAO Inhibitor drugs - Serious Hypertensive Crisis (May Not occur with Levodopa/Carbidopa combinations)

AMATADINE PRODUCTS:

+ Anticholinergics, Alcohol, CNS Stimulants - **May Seriously** increase in side effects of both drugs

SELEGILINE PRODUCTS:

+ Levodopa products - **May Seriously** increase in side effects of latter drug (reduced dosage required)

PERGOLIDE PRODUCTS:

+ Methyldopa, Metoclopropamide, Papaverine, Phenothiazines, Reserpine - May decrease effectiveness former drug

FOOD/NUTRIENT INTERACTIONS:

LEVODOPA PRODUCTS:

+ Pyridoxine products (Vitamin B6) - May decrease effectiveness of former drug (May not with Carbidopa/Sinemet combinations)
+ Protein Rich Diet - May decrease effectiveness of former drug (space protein throughout day with a balanced diet)

SELEGILINE PRODUCTS:

+ Tyramine rich foods (Avocados, some beers/wines, some alcohol "free" beers/wines, figs, some non-fresh fish/meats, fermented sausages, shrimp paste, over-ripe fruits, aged cheese) - May cause **severe** increase in blood pressure
+ Caffeine, chocolate, cottage/cream cheese, yogurt, soy sauce, in large portions or some whiskeys - May cause severe increase in blood pressure

RX LABEL PRECAUTIONS:

May cause drowsiness or discoloration of the urine.
Take prior to and or with food unless pharmacist dictates.

CHART 20 : ANTI-ULCER & H2 BLOCKERS

EXAMPLES:

AXID CARAFATE CIMETIDINE CYTOTEC FAMOTIDINE MISOPROSTOL NIZATIDINE OMEPRAZOLE PEPCID PRILOSEC RANITIDINE SUCRALFATE TAGAMET ZANTAC

INDICATIONS & EFFECTS:

Ulcer, Hypersecretory conditions, and other conditions as determined by physician. H2 blocker effects occur through decreased acid secretion; Prilosec (Omeprazole) also decreases acid pump activity while Cytotec (Misoprostol) increases stomach protection. Sucralfate products bind to ulcer area and promote healing.

DRUG-DISEASE PRECAUTIONS:

Renal or hepatic impairment

DRUG-ALLERGY PRECAUTIONS:

Sensitivity to any ingredients, and prostagladins with Cytotec (Misoprostol)

PRECAUTIONS:

Avoid alcohol, Certain foods, Cigarettes and OTC products may irritate the stomach and decrease effectiveness of this therapy

SIDE EFFECTS: Rare

REPORT: Confusion, Weakness, Irregular heartbeat, Sore throat or fever. Severe diarrhea with Cytotec

MONITOR: Constipation, Vision problems, Rash, Headache, Nausea, Loss of appetite, Decreased libido (Cimetidine)

*** PREGNANCY/NURSING/AGE/STORAGE/ABUSE PRECAUTIONS:**

Inform physician if pregnant/nursing, avoid with Cytotec (Misoprotol). Keep out of children's reach. Disorientation may be more likely in elderly.

Interacting drugs may be used together in some conditions.

DRUG INTERACTIONS FOR: ANTI-ULCER & H2 BLOCKERS

ALL PRODUCTS

+ Antacids - May decrease effects of former drug - Take 1 to 2 hours apart, unless otherwise directed. Avoid Magnesium antacids with Cytotec.
+ Ketoconazole & Enteric Coated Drugs - May decrease effects of latter drug - Take 2 hours apart

SUCRALFATE PRODUCTS: In addition

+ Digoxin, Phenytoin, Tetracyclines, Fluoroquinolones, Vitamins A,D,E,K - May decrease effects of latter drug - Take 2 hours apart

OMEPRAZOLE PRODUCTS: In addition

+ Anticoagulants, Digoxin, Benzodiazepines, Phenytoin - May increase effects of latter drug

CIMETIDINE PRODUCTS: In addition

+ Anticoagulants, Carbamazepine, Lidocaine, Phenytoin, Theophylline, - **May seriously** increase effects of latter drug
+ Alcohol, Benzodiazepines, Beta-blockers, Calcium blockers, Encainide, Flecainide, Hypoglycemics, Procainamide, Quinidine, Valproate, - May increase effects of latter drug
+ Anticholinergics, Cigarettes - May decrease effects of former drug

RANITIDINE PRODUCTS: In addition

+ Fluroquinolones - **May seriously** decrease latter drug - Take 2 hours apart
+ Alcohol, Beta blockers, Hypoglycemics, Phenytoin, Procainamide, Quinidine, Theophylline - May increase effects of latter drug

FOOD/NUTRIENT INTERACTIONS:

+ Iron Products - May decrease effects of latter, except for Cytotec.

RX LABEL PRECAUTIONS:

Avoid alcohol. Take full course of treatment. DO NOT double dose. Take with full glass of water. May take with food.

***Store all medicines out of childrens reach, away from heat and direct sunlight. Discard old/outdated medications. Inform physician(s) or pharmacist of all current medications and any questions that may arise.**

See complete prescribing literature for additional information.

CHART 21 : ARRHYTHMIC AGENTS 1

EXAMPLES:

CARDIOQUIN CIN QUIN DISOPYRAMIDE DURAQUIN NORPACE PROCAINAMIDE PROCAN SR PRONESTYL QUINAGLUTE QUINIDEX QUINIDINE QUINORA

INDICATIONS & EFFECTS:

Antiarrhythmic, Irregular heartbeat and other conditions as determined by physician. Effects occur through decreased heart conduction or velocity thus increasing the refractory period and efficiency of the heart. Quinidine in addition, and efficiency of heart increases B-adrenergic vasodilation effects.

DRUG-DISEASE PRECAUTIONS:

Heart problems, Liver or Renal problems, Breathing problems, Myasthenia gravis or Asthma with Quinidine, Procainamide

DRUG-ALLERGY PRECAUTIONS:

Sensitivity to any ingredients or "Caine" medications with Procainamide

PRECAUTIONS:

Any type of Surgery, Disopyramide - May decrease blood sugar (Hunger, Nausea, Anxiety, Sweating.) Driving alertness, Have frequent check ups, Don't discontinue without checking with physician and avoid alcohol.

SIDE EFFECTS: Rare to Moderate

REPORT: Any change in heart problems, Shortness of breath, Chest pain, Severe dizziness, Rash, Shaking, Vision changes, Urinary changes, Unusual bleeding, Fever or Sore throat

MONITOR: Bitter taste with Quinidine, Dry mouth with Disopyramide, Dizziness, Headache, Nausea, Tiredness

*** PREGNANCY/NURSING/AGE/STORAGE/ABUSE PRECAUTIONS:**

Inform physician if pregnant or nursing. Have frequent check ups. Elderly may be more susceptible to effects

Interacting drugs may be used together in some conditions.

DRUG INTERACTIONS FOR: ARRHYTHMIC AGENTS 1
QUINIDINE PRODUCTS

+ Carbonic Anhydrase Inhibitors, Calcium & Magnesium Antacids, Sodium Bicarbonate, Pimozide, Verapamil - **May seriously** increase effects of former drug
+ Procainamide, Encainide, Quinine - **May seriously** increase effects of latter drug
+ Aspirin, Salicylates, Neuromuscular Blockers - **May seriously** increase side effects of either drug
+ Anticoagulants, Antidepressants Tricyclic, Beta Blockers, Digoxin, Digitoxin, Ketoconazole, Cimetidine, Ranitadine - May increase effects of latter drug
+ Barbiturates, Metoclopramide, Nifedipine, Phenytoin, Primidone, Rifampin - May decrease effects of former drug

PROCAINAMIDE PRODUCTS

+ Amiodarone, Cimetadine, Quinidine, Ranitadine - **May seriously** increase effects of **former** drug
+ Trimethoprim, Bactrim, Septra, Sulfa combinations - **May seriously** increase effects of **former** drug

DISOPYRAMIDE PRODUCTS

+ Calcium Blockers, Erythromycin - **May seriously** increase effects of former drug
+ Anticoagulants, Beta Blockers - May increase effects of latter drug
+ Isosorbide, Nitroglycerin, PETN, Vasodilators - May decrease effects of latter drug
+ Phenytoin, Rifampin - May decrease effects of former drug

FOOD/NUTRIENT INTERACTIONS:

+ Diet - Maintain diet to help assure electrolyte and nutrition balance.

RX LABEL PRECAUTIONS:

Take only as directed with full glass of water. DO NOT double dose.

***Store all medicines out of childrens reach, away from heat and direct sunlight. Discard old/outdated medications.**
Inform physician(s)/pharmacist of all current medications and any questions that may arise.

See complete prescribing literature for additional information.

CHART 22 : ARRHYTHMIC AGENTS 2

EXAMPLES:

AMIODARONE CORDARONE ENCAINIDE ENKAID ETHMOZINE FLECAINIDE MEXILETINE MEXITIL MORICIZINE PROPA-FENONE RYTHMOL TAMBOCOR TOCAINIDE TONOCARD

INDICATIONS & EFFECTS:

Antiarrhythmic, Irregular heartbeat and other conditions as determined by physician. Effects occur through decreased cardiac excitability, conduction velocity or action potential via sodium or calcium channel inhibition with resultant efficiency of heart.

DRUG-DISEASE PRECAUTIONS:

Heart problems, Liver or Renal problems, Breathing problems, Seizures with Mexiletine, Hypo or Hyper Kalemia with Encainide

DRUG-ALLERGY PRECAUTIONS:

Sensitivity to any ingredients or Lidocaine and "Amide" Anesthetics with Flecainide, Mexiletine

PRECAUTIONS:

Any type of Surgery, Driving alertness, Have frequent check ups, Do not discontinue therapy without checking with physician and avoid alcohol.

SIDE EFFECTS: Rare to Moderate

REPORT: Any change in heart problems, Shortness of breath, Chest pain, Severe dizziness, Rash, Shaking, Vision changes, Urinary changes, Unusual bleeding, Fever or Sore throat
MONITOR: Dizziness, Headache, Nausea, Tiredness

*** PREGNANCY/NURSING/AGE/STORAGE/ABUSE PRECAUTIONS:**

Inform physician if pregnant or nursing. Have frequent check ups. Elderly may be more susceptible to effects

Interacting drugs may be used together in some conditions.

DRUG INTERACTIONS FOR: ARRHYTHMIC AGENTS 2

MEXILETINE PRODUCTS

+ Theophyllines - **May seriously** increase effects of latter drug
+ Carbonic Anhydrase Inhibitors, Other Arrhythmics - **May seriously** increase effects of former drug
+ Phenytoin, Rifampin, Smoking - May decrease effects of former drug

ENCAINIDE PRODUCTS

+ Cimetidine, Quinidine, Other Arrhythmics - May increase effects of former drug

AMIODARONE PRODUCTS

+ Anticoagulants, Beta Blockers, Digoxin, Diltiazem, Flecainide, Thiazide Diuretics, Phenytoin, Procainide, Quinidine - May increase effects of latter drug
+ Cholestyramine - **May seriously** decrease effects of former drug
+ Anesthetics, Benzodiazepines - **May seriously** increase effects of former drug
+ Thyroid - May decrease effects of latter drug

TOCAINIDE PRODUCTS

+ Cimetidine - May decrease effects of former drug

FLECAINIDE PRODUCTS

+ Amiodarone, Cimetidine - **May seriously** increase effects of former drug
+ Beta Blockers, Other Arrhythmics - May increase effects of either drug
+ Digoxin - May increase effects of latter drug

PROPAFENONE PRODUCTS

+ Digoxin, Anticoagulants, Other Arrhythmics - May increase effects of latter drug

FOOD/NUTRIENT INTERACTIONS:

+ Diet - Maintain diet to assure electrolyte and nutrition balance

RX LABEL PRECAUTIONS:

Take only as directed with full glass of water. DO NOT double dose.

***Store all medicines out of childrens reach, away from heat and direct sunlight. Discard old/outdated medications.**

Inform physician(s)/pharmacist of all current medications and any questions that may arise.

See complete prescribing literature for additional information.

CHART 23 : BARBITURATES AND RELATED COMBINATIONS

EXAMPLES:

AMYTAL BANCAP BUTABARBITAL BUTALBITAL BUTISOL ESGIC FIORGEN FIORICET FIORINAL LUMINAL MEBARAL NEMBUTAL PHENOBARBITAL SECOBARBITAL SECONAL TUINAL

INDICATIONS & EFFECTS:

Headache, Seizures, Epilepsy, Sedation, and other conditions as determined by physician. Effects occur through CNS depression or GABA agonist action.

DRUG-DISEASE PRECAUTIONS:

Alcoholism, Asthma, Breathing problems, Kidney or Liver problems, Drug dependency history or abuse, Mental depression

DRUG-ALLERGY PRECAUTIONS:

Sensitivity to any ingredients

PRECAUTIONS:

Alcohol and any other CNS depressants, Drug dependency history or abuse, Decreased respiration, Drowsiness, Unsteadiness, Possible withdrawal (Nervousness, Mental changes, Fast heartbeat, Confusion, Sleeplessness) - Dosage should be decreased gradually over a 2-6 week period. Long term use may bea habit forming with resultant anxiety, confusion, decreased memory and poor judgement.

SIDE EFFECTS: Moderate

REPORT: See Also Precautions. Allergic reactions, Breathing problems, Hallucinations, Hangover effects, Irritability, Severe mental depression or confusion, Severe drowsiness, Skin discoloration, Unusual weakness or bleeding

MONITOR: Dizziness, Lightheadedness, Nausea, Sleeplessness

*** PREGNANCY/NURSING/AGE/STORAGE/ABUSE PRECAUTIONS:**

Inform physician if pregnant or nursing. Best avoided if pregnant unless otherwise directed by physician. Elderly and children may be more sensitive to effects. May be habit forming. Avoid long term use unless otherwise directed.

Interacting drugs may be used together in some conditions.

DRUG INTERACTIONS FOR: BARBITURATES AND RELATED COMBINATIONS

+ Alcohol, Antihistimines, Anti-Anxiety Agents, Hypnotics, Narcotics, Sedatives - May increase side effects of either drug
+ Anticoagulants, Beta Blockers, Carbamazepine, Oral contraceptives, Guanfacine, Haloperidol, Metrodazole, Phenothiazine, Theophyllines, Tetracycline - **May seriously** decrease effects of latter drug
+ Antidepressants Tricyclic, Steroids, Cyclosporine, Digitoxin, Quinidine, Verapamil - May decrease effect of latter drug
+ Chloramphenicol, Flu vaccine, Valproate - May increase effects of former drug

FOOD/NUTRIENT INTERACTIONS:

+ Ascorbic Acid (Vitamin C) - May decrease effects of latter

RX LABEL PRECAUTIONS:

May cause drowsiness - Use caution driving and operating machinery. Avoid alcohol. DO NOT double dose.

***Store all medicines out of childrens reach, away from heat and direct sunlight. Discard old/outdated medications.**
Inform physician(s)/pharmacist of all current medications and any questions that may arise.

See complete prescribing literature for additional information.

CHART 24 : BETA BLOCKERS

EXAMPLES:

ACEBUTOLOL ATENOLOL CARTEOLOL CARTROL CORGARD CORZIDE INDERAL INDERIDE LABETALOL LEVATOL LOPRESSOR METOPROLOL NADALOL NORMODYNE NORMOZIDE PENBUTALOL PINDOLOL PROPRANOLOL SECTRAL TENORMIN TENORETIC TIMOLIDE TOPROL XL TRANDATE VISKEN

INDICATIONS & EFFECTS:

Angina, Certain cardiac or blood pressure conditions, Headache, Glaucoma, Anxiety and other conditions as determined by physician. Effects occur through blocking beta-1 receptors (cardioselective) in the heart and/or beta-2 receptors, resluting in decreased angina blood pressure and arrhythmia. (Nonselective), ISA effects occur if B-adrenergic stimulation occurs simultaneously, i.e. Pindolol.

DRUG-DISEASE PRECAUTIONS:

Cardiac failure, Heart block or rate less than 48 beats per minute, Asthma, Emphysema, Diabetes, Hepatic or Renal problems, Depression Psoriasis, Hyperthyroidism, or Pheochromocytoma

DRUG-ALLERGY PRECAUTIONS:

Sensitivity to any ingredients, Allergies

PRECAUTIONS:

Avoid alcohol, Gradual dosage decrease may be required if discontinuing, Check with physician, Surgery, Diabetes, Overexertion

SIDE EFFECTS: Rare to Moderate

REPORT: Allergy, Skin rash, Joint pain, Irregular heartbeat, Breathing problems, Chest pain, Confusion, Depression, Fever or sore throat, Cold in hands or feet, Sweating, Extreme weakness

MONITOR: Anxiety, Constipation or Diarrhea, Decreased libido, Drowsiness, Nausea, Itching, Numbness, Stuffy nose, Restlessness

*** PREGNANCY/NURSING/AGE/STORAGE/ABUSE PRECAUTIONS:**

Best avoided if pregnant or nursing if directed by physician, Elderly may be more susceptible to effects

Interacting drugs may be used together in some conditions.

DRUG INTERACTIONS FOR: BETA BLOCKERS

+ Diabetic Agents and Insulin (Beta-1 Blockers, Atenolol, Betaxolol, Metropolol are less likely to interact), Calcium Blockers, Clonidine, Guanabenz, Reserpine, MAO Inhibitors (up to 14 days after therapy with MAOI) **May seriously** increase effects of latter drug
+ Cocaine, CNS Stimulants, Decongestants. OTC diet aids - **May seriously** decrease effects of former drug
+ Theophylline, Xanthines, Bronchodilators (Beta-1 Blockers less likely to interact) - **May seriously** decrease effects of latter drug
+ Alcohol, Anesthetics inhalation, Nitroglycerin, Phenothiazines, Cimetidine, Ranitadine - May increase effects of former drug

FOOD/NUTRIENT INTERACTIONS:

+ Food Allergies or Stinging insects - May increase severity of allergic reaction

RX LABEL PRECAUTIONS:

May cause drowsiness. Avoid alcohol. May take with food.

***Store all medicines out of childrens reach, away from heat and direct sunlight. Discard old/outdated medications.**
Inform physician(s)/pharmacist of all current medications and any questions that may arise.

See complete prescribing literature for additional information.

CHART 25 : BRONCHODILATORS

EXAMPLES:

ADRENALIN ALBUTEROL ALUPENT ATROVENT BRETHAIRE BRETHINE BRONKOSOL EPINEPHRINE ISOPROTERENOL ISUPREL MAXAIR MEDIHALER METAPROTERENOL NORISODRINE PROVENTIL SUS-PHRINE TERBUTALINE TORNALATE VENTOLIN

INDICATIONS & EFFECTS:

Asthma, Bronchitis, Emphysema, Pulmonary Disease, Allergic reactions, Anaphylactic shock, Hypotension, Cardiac conditions, Congestion, reactions and other conditions. Beta-agonist effects occur through stimulating beta-2 adrenergic receptors to relax bronchial smooth muscle. Epinephrine and Metaproterenol also may decrease histamine.

DRUG-DISEASE PRECAUTIONS:

Cardiovascular Disease, Convulsive disorders, Diabetes, Hyperthyroidism, Pheochromocytoma, Shock

DRUG-ALLERGY PRECAUTIONS:

Sensitivity to any ingredients, decongestants and/or CNS stimulants. Some preparations may contain sulfites.

PRECAUTIONS:

Increased heart rate or difficulty in breathing. Do not use more than pre-scribed dosage. Daily use may indicate another drug may be needed to help control condition.

SIDE EFFECTS: Rare to Moderate

REPORT: Chest pain, Increased blood pressure, Changes in sleeplessness, breathing, Severe dizziness or headache, Irregular heartbeat, Blurred vision, Excessive nervousness, Severe weakness

MONITOR: Coughing, Lightheadedness, Dry mouth, Flushing, Nausea, Restlessness, Sensory changes

*** PREGNANCY/NURSING/AGE/STORAGE/ABUSE PRECAUTIONS:**

Inform physician if pregnant/nursing, may need to discontinue certain medications. Exercise extreme caution in infants and children. Epinephrine should be stored in the refrigerator.

Interacting drugs may be used together in some conditions.

DRUG INTERACTIONS FOR: BRONCHODILATORS

+ Ergot - **Serious** vasoconstriction with ephedrine and epinephrine
+ Beta blockers - **May seriously** decrease effectiveness of former drug, less severe with Beta-1 blockers
+ Digoxin, Thiazides - May increase side effects of latter drug
+ Anesthetics, Levodopa, Antidepressants, MAOI's - **May seriously** increase side effects of former drug
+ Nitrates, Vasodilators - May decrease effectiveness of latter drug
+ Cocaine, Decongestants, CNS stimulants, Thyroids, Theophyllines, Xanthines and Caffeine - **May seriously** increase the side effects of either drug

FOOD/NUTRIENT INTERACTIONS:

+ Large amounts of Soda, Tea and or coffee - May cause serious increase in side effects of either

RX LABEL PRECAUTIONS:

Use only as directed. Do NOT double dose. For inhalation products, shake canister well. For oral tablets, do not crush.

***Store all medicines out of childrens reach, away from heat and direct sunlight. Discard old/outdated medications.**
Inform physician(s)/pharmacist of all current medications and any questions that may arise.

See complete prescribing literature for additional information.

CHART 26 : CALCIUM CHANNEL BLOCKERS

EXAMPLES:

ADALAT BEPRIDIL CALAN CARDENE CARDIZEM DILTIAZEM DYNACIRC FELODIPINE ISOPTIN ISRADIPINE NICARDIPINE NIFEDIPINE NIMODIPINE NIMOTOP PLENDIL PROCARDIA VASCOR VERAPAMIL VERELAN

INDICATIONS & EFFECTS:

Angina, Irregular Heartbeat, Hypertension, and other conditions determined by physician. Effects occur through decreased calcium transport in myocardial cells and vascular smooth muscle thus decreasing arterial pressure, vascular resistance with resultant vasodilitation and improved cardiac output.

DRUG-DISEASE PRECAUTIONS:

Caution in other Cardiovascular, Renal and Hepatic Diseases, Severe hypotension, Myocardial infarction

DRUG-ALLERGY PRECAUTIONS:

Sensitivity to any ingredient

PRECAUTIONS:

Check pulse, Have frequent check ups, May need to taper dose if discontinuing therapy with physician. Exercise caution returning to more normal activities, take it slowly.

SIDE EFFECTS: Rare to Moderate

REPORT: Allergic reaction, Rash, Chest pain, Faintness, Heart problems, Swelling or Vision problem

MONITOR: Constipation, Dizziness, Nausea, Headache, Swelling, Tiredness

*** PREGNANCY/NURSING/AGE/STORAGE/ABUSE PRECAUTIONS:**

Best avoided if pregnant or nursing unless otherwise directed by physician. Protect drug from direct sunlight. Elderly may be more sensitive to effects

Interacting drugs may be used together in some conditions.

DRUG INTERACTIONS FOR: CALCIUM CHANNEL BLOCKERS

ALL PRODUCTS

+ Antiarrythmics, Disopyramide - **May seriously** increase effects of either drug
+ Alcohol, Beta-blockers, Caffeine, Carbamazepine, Cyclosporine, Digitalis, Diabetic Agents, Quinidine, Alpha Adrenergic Blockers, Prazocin, Lithium, Terfenadine, Theophyllines - **May seriously** increase effects of latter drug
+ Cimetidine - **May seriously** increase effects of former drug
+ Anticonvulsants, Barbiturates, Rifampin, Sulfinpyrazone, CNS Stimulants, Decongestants, Non steroidal Anti-inflammatories - May decrease effects of former drug

VERAPAMIL & DILTIAZEM PRODUCTS - In addition

+ Beta Blockers, Digoxin - **May seriously** increase effects of latter drug
+ Valproate- may increase effects of latter drug.

FOOD/NUTRIENT INTERACTIONS:

+ Calcium Supplements in large dosages - May decrease effects of former drug
+ Grapefruit juice - May increase effects of former drug - Take drug with water

RX LABEL PRECAUTIONS:

Take only as directed with full glass of water. May take with food.

***Store all medicines out of childrens reach, away from heat and direct sunlight. Discard old/outdated medications.**
Inform physician(s)/pharmacist of all current medications and any questions that may arise.

See complete prescribing literature for additional information.

CHART 27 : CARBONIC ANHYDRASE INHIBITORS

EXAMPLES:

ACETAZOLAMIDE DARANIDE DIAMOX DICHLORPHEN-AMID METHAZOLAMIDE NEPTAZANE

INDICATIONS & EFFECTS:

Glaucoma, Edema, and other conditions as determined by physician. Effects occur through inhibiting the carbonic anhydrase enzyme, thus decreasing hydrogen and bicarbonate ions producing diruresis and lower pressure.

DRUG-DISEASE PRECAUTIONS:

Breathing problems, Diabetes, Liver or Kidney problems, Pregnancy, Electrolyte Imbalance, Adrenal problems

DRUG-ALLERGY PRECAUTIONS:

Sulfa Allergy, Thiazide or Diabetic Agent Allergy, or sensitivity to any ingredient

PRECAUTIONS:

Frequent check ups, DO NOT double dose, Acidosis, Low Potassium (Muscle Cramps, Weakness, Irregular heartbeat or breathing) or Low Sodium (Mental changes, Low blood pressure, Irregular heartbeat), DO NOT abruptly stop taking unless directed, May increase sun sensitivity - Use sunscreen when outside for extended periods

SIDE EFFECTS: Moderate

REPORT: Breathing problems, Unusual bleeding, Sore throat, Fever or Tiredness, Urinary problems, Confusion, Dry mouth, Muscle cramps, Irregular heartbeat, Mental changes

MONITOR: Constipation or Diarrhea, Drowsiness, Headache, Loss of appetite, Mental taste, Numbness, Irritability, Increase in blood sugar

*** PREGNANCY/NURSING/AGE/STORAGE/ABUSE PRECAUTIONS:**

Avoid in pregnancy or nursing. Elderly may be more susceptible to effects

Interacting drugs may be used together in some conditions.

DRUG INTERACTIONS FOR: CARBONIC ANHYDRASE INHIBITORS

+ Diuretics, Quinidine, CNS Stimulants, Decongestants, Salicylates, Mexiletine - **May seriously** increase effects of latter drug
+ Digoxin, Steroids, Ciprofloxacin, Phenytoin - May increase effects of latter drug
+ Diabetic Agents, Insulin, Lithium - May decrease effects of latter drug

FOOD/NUTRIENT INTERACTIONS:

+ Low Sodium or low Potassium Diet - **May seriously** increase side effects of former drug. Maintain balanced diet.

RX LABEL PRECAUTIONS:

Take with food and full glass of water. DO NOT double dose.

***Store all medicines out of childrens reach, away from heat and direct sunlight. Discard old/outdated medications.**
Inform physician(s)/pharmacist of all current medications and any questions that may arise.

See complete prescribing literature for additional information.

CHART 28 : CEPHALOSPORINS

EXAMPLES:

CECLOR CEFACLOR CEFADROXIL CEFIZOX CEFTIN CEFPROZIL CEFZIL CEPHRADINE CEPTAZ CLAFORAN DURICEF FORTAZ KEFLET KEFLEX KEFTAB MEFOXIN MONOCID MOXAM ROCEPHIN SUPRAX TAZICEF VELOSEF ZINACEF

INDICATIONS & EFFECTS:

Antibiotics for infections i.e. Upper and lower respiratory tract, Bone and joint infections, Soft tissue, Gastrointestinal, Genitourinary, Skin, Otitis media and other conditions as determined by your physician. Effects occur through bacteriocidal action on bacteria cell wall synthesis.

DRUG-DISEASE PRECAUTIONS:

Bleeding disorders (may decrease Vitamin K activity), Gastrointestinal problems, Renal function impairment.

DRUG-ALLERGY PRECAUTIONS:

Sensitivity to Penicillins, Cephalosporin, Penicillamine

PRECAUTIONS:

Avoid alcohol while on therapy, Have frequent check ups, Superinfections, lab test for long term therapy, Diabetics - May cause false urine test results with Copper Sulfite tests.

SIDE EFFECTS: Rare to Moderate

Report: Severe diarrhea, Breathing problems, Dizziness, Skin rash, Itching, Cramps, Bloating, Unusual bleeding or blood in urine, Vaginal infections

Monitor: Mild diarrhea, Nausea, Vomiting, Sore mouth

*** PREGNANCY/NURSING/AGE/STORAGE/ABUSE PRECAUTIONS:**

Inform physician if pregnant/nursing, most liquid oral preparations may require refrigeration - Do Not Freeze, and Shake Well.

Interacting drugs may be used together in some conditions.

DRUG INTERACTIONS FOR: CEPHALOSPORINS
ALL PRODUCTS

+ Alcohol, Aminoglycosides, Anticoagulants, Heparin, Loop Diuretics, Vancomycin - **May seriously** increase effects of latter drug
+ Oral contraceptives (estrogen) - May decrease effectiveness of latter drug
+ Probenecid - May increase effects of former drug

MOXALACTAM PRODUCTS: In addition

+ Aspirin, Salicylates, Heparin - **May seriously** increase side effects of either drug

FOOD/NUTRIENT INTERACTIONS:

+ Food - Maintain balanced diet to aid in recovery.

RX LABEL PRECAUTIONS:

Take with full glass of water on empty stomach if possible. May take with food if upsetting to stomach. Take full course of treatment unless otherwise directed.

***Store all medicines out of childrens reach, away from heat and direct sunlight. Discard old/outdated medications.**
Inform physician(s)/pharmacist of all current medications and any questions that may arise.

See complete prescribing literature for additional information.

CHART 29 : CHOLESTEROL AGENTS

EXAMPLES:

ATROMID-S CHOLESTYRAMINE CLOFIBRATE COLESTID COLESTIPOL GEMFIBROZIL LOPID LORELCO LOVASTATIN MEVACOR NIACIN NICOBID NICOLAR PRAVACHOL PRAVASTATIN PROBUCOL QUESTRAN SIMVASTATIN VITAMIN B3 ZOCOR

INDICATIONS & EFFECTS:

Hyperlipidemia and other conditions. Powders' binding action reduces cholesterol. HMG-CoA reductace inhibitors and others reduce formation of cholesterol.

DRUG-DISEASE PRECAUTIONS:

Certain Convulsant disorders, Alcoholism, Liver or Renal problems,
In addition; Clofibrate & Gemfibrozol - Gallbladder problems
Lovastatin, Pravastatin, Simvastatin - Surgery, Metabolic disorders, Severe infection, Hypotension, Seizures
Probucol - Arrhythmias, Hypokalemia; & Niacin - Ulcer

DRUG-ALLERGY PRECAUTIONS:

Sensitivity to any ingredients

PRECAUTIONS:

Maintain prescribed balanced diet, Have frequent check ups, mix powders as directed, Avoid smoking

SIDE EFFECTS: Rare to Moderate

REPORT: Vision problems, Fever or chills, Muscular aches and pain, Urinary problems, Unusual weakness, Severe dizziness, Jaundice

MONITOR: Nausea, Dizziness, Joint pain, Increased thirst/Urination, Gas, Rash, Numbness, Niacin Flushing: Take with food if no relief after a week, may try one aspirin tablet 30 minutes before a meal and Niacin dose unless otherwise directed

*** PREGNANCY/NURSING/AGE/STORAGE/ABUSE PRECAUTIONS:**

Best avoided if pregnant or nursing (Except Niacin). Elderly may be more sensitive to effects. Not recommended in children less than two.

Interacting drugs may be used together in some conditions.

DRUG INTERACTIONS FOR: CHOLESTEROL AGENTS

CHOLESTYRAMINE and COLESTIPOL PRODUCTS

- + Amiodarone, Antibiotics, Anticoagulants, Digitalis, Diuretics, Other Cholesterol Agents, Beta-Blockers, Thyroid - May decrease effect of latter drug (Take 4 to 6 hours apart unless otherwise directed)

CLOFIBRATE PRODUCTS

- + Anticoagulants, Diabetic Oral Agents, Furosemide - **May seriously** increase effects of latter drug
- + Contraceptives, Probucol, Rifampin - **May seriously** decrease effects of former drug
- + Probenecid - **May seriously** increase effects of former drug

GEMFIBROZIL PRODUCTS

- + Lovastatin - **May seriously** increase side effects of latter drug
- + Diabetic Agents and Insulin - May decrease effects of latter drug

LOVASTATIN, PRAVASTATIN, SIMVASTATIN PRODUCTS

- + Erythromycin, Cyclosporine, Gemfibrozil, Niacin - **May seriously** increase side effects of former drug
- + Anticoagulants, (Simvastatin + Digoxin) - May increase effects of latter drug

NIACIN PRODUCTS (B3)

- + Chenodiol - May decrease effects of latter drug
- + Lovastatin - May increase side effects of latter drug

PROBUCOL PRODUCTS

- + Chenodiol, Clofibrate - **May seriously** decrease effects of latter drug
- + Anti-Arrhythmics, Digoxin - May increase effects of latter drug

FOOD/NUTRIENT INTERACTIONS:

- + Diet - Maintain well balanced diet as first defense to high cholesterol

RX LABEL PRECAUTIONS:

Take with food unless otherwise directed. Avoid alcohol & smoking.

***Store all medicines out of childrens reach, away from heat and direct sunlight. Discard old/outdated medications. Inform physician(s) or pharmacist of all current medications and any questions that may arise.**

See complete prescribing literature for additional information.

CHART 30 : CNS STIMULANTS

EXAMPLES:

ADIPEX-P AMPHETAMINE DEXEDRINE DEXTROAMPHETAMINE DIDREX DIETHYLPROPION FASTIN IONAMIN MAZANOR METHYLPHENIDATE PEMOLINE PHENDIMETRAZINE PHENTERMINE PLEGINE PONDIMIN PRELU-2 RITALIN SANOREX TENUATE TEPANIL

INDICATIONS & EFFECTS:

Appetite suppressant, Narcolepsy, Temporary aid in weight loss program, and other conditions as determined by physician. Effects occur through CNS stimulation.

DRUG-DISEASE PRECAUTIONS:

Anxiety, Arrythmia, Cardiovascular disease, Hypertension, Hyperthyroidism, Glaucoma, Drug dependency history or abuse.

DRUG-ALLERGY PRECAUTIONS:

Sensitivity to any of the ingredients or other sympathomimetics, i.e. Isoproterenol, Epinephrine, Adrenalin, Terbutaline.

PRECAUTIONS:

Drug dependency history. Use caution if taking other CNS stimulants, caffeine or appetite suppressants - May result in mental changes or disorientation; possible sleeplessness if taken late in the day. Possibility of withdrawal.

SIDE EFFECTS: Rare to Moderate

REPORT: Severe increase in Blood pressure, Diarrhea, Headache, Irregular heartbeat, Mood or mental changes, Shortness of breath, Severe nausea.

MONITOR: Difficulty in sleeping, Fever, Vision problems, Increase in blood pressure, Decreased libido, Unsteadiness.

*** PREGNANCY/NURSING/AGE/STORAGE/ABUSE PRECAUTIONS:**

Inform physician if pregnant/nursing - Best avoided in pregnancy & may need to discontinue nursing. Mood changes, particularly in children; overdose more dangerous in children; monitor response in elderly. May be habit forming. Avoid long term use unless otherwise directed.

Interacting drugs may be used together in some conditions.

DRUG INTERACTIONS FOR: CNS STIMULANTS

+ Digoxin, Anesthetics - **May seriously** increase side effects of former drug
+ Antidepressants, Anticholinergics - May cause increase in side effects of former drug
+ Beta blockers, Guanadrel, Guanethidine - **May seriously** decrease the effectiveness of latter drug
+ Alcohol, Bronchodilators, Caffeine, Cocaine, MAO inhibitors, Theophyllines, Thyroids -**May seriously** increase side effects of either drug
+ Insulin & Diabetic agents - May decrease effectiveness of latter drug
+ Cough/cold remedies - May increase effects of either drug since many contain decongestant ingredients which are closely related to this group (read labels for all ingredients), or check with your pharmacist or physician.

FOOD/NUTRIENT INTERACTIONS:

+ Large consumption of coffee, soda and tea - May increase effects of either

RX LABEL PRECAUTIONS:

Take only as directed by physician. DO NOT double dose.

***Store all medicines out of childrens reach, away from heat and direct sunlight. Discard old/outdated medications.**
Inform physician(s)/pharmacist of all current medications and any questions that may arise.

See complete prescribing literature for additional information.

CHART 31 : COUGH & COLD & EXPECTORANTS

EXAMPLES: Refer to drug names in index.
ANTIHISTAMINE INGREDIENTS (BROMPHENIRAMINE CHLORPHENIRAMINE DIPHENHYDRAMINE PHENINDAMINE PROMETHAZINE PYRILAMINE) See Also CHART 17.
DECONGESTANTINGREDIENTS (PHENYLPROPANOLAMINE PPA PSEUDOPHEDRINE PHENYLEPHRINE) See Also CHART 33.
EXPECTORANTS (GUIAFENESIN IODIDES) Refer to this CHART.

INDICATIONS & EFFECTS:
Productive cough, Cold symptoms, and other conditions as determined by physician. Expectorant effects result in loosening mucus secretions. See above charts for additional effects.

DRUG-DISEASE PRECAUTIONS:
Antihistamines: Acute asthma, Glaucoma, Urinary conditions
Decongestants: Arrhythmias, Heart conditions, Diabetes, Glaucoma, Hypertension
Iodides: Hyperthyroid disease, Pregnancy, Acne

DRUG-ALLERGY PRECAUTIONS:
Sensitivity to any ingredients in product or combination

PRECAUTIONS:
Antihistamines: Avoid alcohol, Drowsiness, Sun sensitivity, Other CNS depressants
Decongestants: Sleeplessness, Other CNS stimulants and caffeine
Iodide Expectorants: Thyroid function with long term therapy

SIDE EFFECTS: Moderate
REPORT: Allergic reactions, Swelling, Unusual bleeding, Change in heart rate, Confusion, Shortness of breath, Change in blood pressure, Severe drowsiness, Headache, Mood changes
Iodides in addition: Chills, Fever, Metallic taste, Sore throat, cold sensitivity
MONITOR: Drowsiness, Sleeplessness, Dizziness, Dry mouth

* **PREGNANCY/NURSING/AGE/STORAGE/ABUSE PRECAUTIONS:**
Best avoided if pregnant or nursing unless otherwise directed. Elderly may be more sensitive to effects. Iodides should be avoided in pregnancy or nursing and children unless otherwise directed.

Interacting drugs may be used together in some conditions.

DRUG INTERACTIONS FOR: COUGH & COLD & EXPECTORANTS
ANTIHISTIMINE & DECONGESTANT INGREDIENTS

+ Alcohol, Antidepressants, CNS Depressants, Barbiturates, Antianxiety drugs, Cough and cold remedies, Narcotics, Muscle relaxants - May cause increase in side effects of either drug
+ Digoxin, Anesthetics - May cause increase in side effects of former drug
+ Anticholinergics - May cause serious increase in side effects of latter drug
+ Beta Blockers, Guanadrel, Guanethidine - May cause serious decrease in effectiveness of latter drug
+ Brochodilators, Cocaine, MAO Inhibitors, Theophyllines - May cause serious increase in side effects of either drug
  Insulin - May decrease effects of latter drug

IODIDES & IODINATED PRODUCTS - In addition

+ Lithium, Antithyroids - **May seriously** increase side effects of former drug

FOOD/NUTRIENT INTERACTIONS:

+ Large consumption of coffee, soda and tea - May increase effects of either

RX LABEL PRECAUTIONS:

Avoid alcohol. May cause drowsiness. Do Not double dose.

***Store all medicines out of childrens reach, away from heat and direct sunlight. Discard old/outdated medications.**
Inform physician(s)/pharmacist of all current medications and any questions that may arise.

See complete prescribing literature for additional information.

CHART 32 : COUGH, COLD, & SUPPRESSANTS

EXAMPLES: Refer to drug names in index.

ANTIHISTAMINES (BROMPHENIRAMINE CHLORPHENIRAMINE DIPHENHYDRAMINE PHENINDAMINE PROMETHAZINE PYRILAMINE) See Also CHART 17.

DECONGESTANTS (PHENYLPROPANOLAMINE PSEUDOPHEDRINE PHENYLEPHRINE) See Also CHART 33.

SUPPRESSANTS (CODEINE HYDROCODONE)
See Also CHART 51.

SUPPRESSANTS (DEXTROMETHORPHAN) Refer to this section

INDICATIONS & EFFECTS:

Dry hacking cough, Cold symptoms, and other conditions. Suppressant effects result in decreased cough reflex.

DRUG-DISEASE PRECAUTIONS:

Antihistamines: Acute asthma, Glaucoma, Urinary and prostatic conditions

Decongestants: Arrhythmias, Heart condition, Diabetes, Glaucoma, Hypertension

Codeine Hydrocodone: Alcoholism, Drug abuse, Heart and breathing problems, Liver disease

Dextromethorphan: Asthma, CNS depression

DRUG-ALLERGY PRECAUTIONS:

Sensitivity to any ingredients in product or combination

PRECAUTIONS:

Antihistamines: Avoid alcohol, Drowsiness, Sun sensitivity, Other CNS depressants

Decongestants: Sleeplessness, Other CNS stimulants and caffeine

Suppressants: Drowsiness, CNS depressants, Respiration

SIDE EFFECTS: Moderate

REPORT: Allergic reactions, Swelling, Unusual bleeding, Change in heart rate, Confusion, Shortness of breath, Change in blood pressure, Severe drowsiness, Headache, Mood changes

MONITOR: Drowsiness, Sleeplessness, Dizziness, Dry mouth

*** PREGNANCY/NURSING/AGE/STORAGE/ABUSE PRECAUTIONS:**

Best avoided if pregnant or nursing unless otherwise directed. Elderly may be more sensitive to effects.

Interacting drugs may be used together in some conditions.

DRUG INTERACTIONS FOR: COUGH & COLD & SUPPRESSANTS
ANTIHISTIMINE & DECONGESTANT INGREDIENTS

+ Alcohol, Antidepressants, CNS Depressants, Barbiturates, Antianxiety drugs, Cough and cold remedies, Narcotics, Muscle relaxants - May cause increase in side effects of either drug
+ Digoxin, Anesthetics - May cause increase in side effects of former drug
+ Anticholinergics - May cause serious increase in side effects of latter drug
+ Beta Blockers, Guanadrel, Guanethidine - May cause **serious** decrease in effectiveness of latter drug
+ Brochodilators, Cocaine, MAO Inhibitors, Theophyllines - May cause **serious** increase in side effects of either drug
+ Insulin - May decrease effects of latter drug

SUPPRESSANTS containing CODEINE, HYDROCODONE

+ Alcohol, Antidepressants, Anxiety Agents, Anticholinergics, Antihistamines, Barbiturates, Hypnotics, Neuromuscular
+ Blockers, Sedatives - **May seriously** increase side effects of either drug
+ Antihypertensives, Diuretics, Guanethidine - May increase side effects of latter drug
+ Narcotic Antagonist - **May seriously** increase withdrawal complications in dependent or abusive patient

SUPPRESSANTS containing DEXTROMETHORPHEN

+ Alcohol, Antidepressants, Antianxiety Agents, Anticholinergics, Antihistamines, Barbiturates, Hypnotics, Neuromuscular Blockers, Sedatives - **May seriously** increase side effects of either drug
+ MAO Inhibitors - **May seriously** increase side effects of latter drug

FOOD/NUTRIENT INTERACTIONS:

+ Large consumption of coffee, soda and tea - May increase effects of either

RX LABEL PRECAUTIONS:

Avoid alcohol. May cause drowsiness. Do Not double dose.

***Store all medicines out of childrens reach, away from heat and direct sunlight. Discard old/outdated medications. Inform physician(s) or pharmacist of all current medications and any questions that may arise.**

See complete prescribing literature for additional information.

CHART 33 : DECONGESTANTS & OTC DIET AIDS

EXAMPLES:

ACUTRIM AFRINOL DEXATRIM NOVAFED PHENYLPROPANOLAMIN PPA PROPADRINE PROPAGEST PSEUDOEPHEDRINE SUDAFED

INDICATIONS & EFFECTS:

Nasal congestion, Sinus headache, Allergies, Aid in weight loss program and other conditions. Effects occur through vasoconstriction decreased swelling and CNS stimulation with diet aids.

DRUG-DISEASE PRECAUTIONS:

Arrythmia, Cardiovascular disease, Diabetes, Hypertension, Hyperthyroidism, Glaucoma, Drug dependency history.

DRUG-ALLERGY PRECAUTIONS:

Sensitivity to any of the ingredients or other sympathomimetics, i.e. Amphetamines, Isoproternol, Epinephrine, Adrenalin, Terbutaline.

PRECAUTIONS:

Use caution if taking other CNS stimulants, caffeine or appetite suppressants - May result in mental changes or disorientation; possible sleeplessness if taken late in the day.

SIDE EFFECTS: Moderate

REPORT: Severe increase in Blood pressure, Headache, Mood or mental changes, Shortness of breath, Severe nausea.
MONITOR: Difficulty in sleeping, Fever, Vision problems, Increase in blood pressure.

*** PREGNANCY/NURSING/AGE/STORAGE/ABUSE PRECAUTIONS:**

Inform physician if pregnant/nursing - May need to discontinue nursing; mood changes, particularly in children; overdose more dangerous in children; monitor response in elderly.

Interacting drugs may be used together in some conditions.

DRUG INTERACTIONS FOR: DECONGESTANTS & OTC DIET AIDS

+ Digoxin, Anesthetics - **May seriously** increase the side effects of former drug
+ Antidepressants, Anticholinergics - May cause increase in side effects of former drug
+ Beta blockers, Guanadrel, Guanethidine - **May seriously** decrease the effectiveness of latter drug
+ Bronchodilators, Caffeine, CNS stimulants, Cocaine, MAO inhibitors, Theophyllines, Thyroids - **May seriously** increase the side effects of either drug
+ Insulin - May decrease effectiveness of latter drug
+ Cough and cold remedies - May increase effects of either drug since many contain ingredients of this group (read labels for all ingredients), or check with your pharmacist or physician.

FOOD/NUTRIENT INTERACTIONS:

+ Large consumption of coffee, soda and tea - May increase effects of either

RX LABEL PRECAUTIONS:

Take only as directed by physician. DO NOT double dose.

***Store all medicines out of childrens reach, away from heat and direct sunlight. Discard old/outdated medications.**
Inform physician(s)/pharmacist of all current medications and any questions that may arise.

See complete prescribing literature for additional information.

CHART 34 : DIABETIC AGENTS & INSULINS

EXAMPLES:

ACETOHEXAMIDE CHLORPROPAMIDE DIABETA DIABINESE DYMELOR GLIPIZIDE GLUCOTROL GLYBURIDE GLYNASE HUMULIN R,N,L,U INSULIN BEEF INSULIN LENTE INSULIN NPH INSULIN PORK INSULIN U MICRONASE MIXTARD NOVOLIN L,N,R ORINASE TOLAZAMIDE TOLBUTAMIDE TOLINASE

INDICATIONS & EFFECTS:

Diabetes. Effects through stimulating or replacing insulin.

DRUG-DISEASE PRECAUTIONS:

Hypo or Hyperthyroidism, Renal problems, Severe fever or Infect-Ions, Oral Agents in addition, Trauma, Thyroid or Liver problems

DRUG-ALLERGY PRECAUTIONS:

Sensitivity to any ingredients. Beef or Pork for some insulins. For oral medications - sensitivity to Thiazide Diuretics, Carbonic Anhydrase Inhibitors or Sulfa drugs

PRECAUTIONS:

Have frequent check ups. Follow diet and avoid alcohol. Tests for blood/urine glucose, May cause sun sensitivity - Use sun-screen outside. **Hyperglycemia** (Increased blood sugar - Ketoacidosis, Dry skin and mouth, Drowsiness, Nausea or vomiting, Increased thirst and urination, Breathing problems, Breath odor, Loss of appetite. **Hypoglycemia** (Decresed blood sugar - Cool skin, Sweating, Nervousness, Drowsiness, Headaches, Nausea, Increased hunger, Fatigue, Increased pulse, Vision problems - May use sugar/candy to correct.

SIDE EFFECTS: Rare to Moderate

REPORT: Hypo or Hyperglycemia as noted in precautions, Oral Agents in addition, Swelling, Breathing problems, Muscle cramps, Unusual sore throat, Fever, Tiredness, Urinary problems **MONITOR:** Constipation, Diarrhea, Minor drowsiness, Nausea, Changes in taste

*** PREGNANCY/NURSING/AGE/STORAGE/ABUSE PRECAUTIONS:**

Oral Agents. Best avoided in pregnancy or nursing unless otherwise directed. Elderly may be more sensitive to effects. Store in refrigerator. DO NOT freeze, Shake gently. DO NOT use insulin which sticks to sides of vial.

Interacting drugs may be used together in some conditions.

DRUG INTERACTIONS FOR: DIABETIC AGENTS AND INSULINS
ALL PRODUCTS

+ Alcohol, Beta Blockers, Guanethidine, MAO Inhibitors - **May seriously** increase effects of former drug
+ Ace Inhibitors, Anabolic and Androgenic Steroids, Non steroidal Anti-inflammatories, Salicylates in large doses - May increase effects of former drug
+ Steroids - **May seriously** decrease effects of former drug by increasing blood glucose
+ Calcium Channel Blockers, Carbonic Anhydrase Inhibitors, Thiazide and Loop Diuretics, Thyroid, Phenytoin, Triamterene - May decrease effects of former drug by increasing blood glucose

ORAL AGENTS - In addition

+ Anticoagulants, Antiulcer H2 Blockers, Chloramphenicol, Clofibrate, Sulfas, Ketoconazole, Miconazole, Sulfinpyrazone - **May seriously** increase effects of former drug
+ Rifampin - **May seriously** decrease effects of former drug

INSULIN INJECTABLE AGENTS - In addition

+ Nicotine gum or patch, Lobeline, Nicotine smoking - May increase effects of former drug

FOOD/NUTRIENT INTERACTIONS:

+ Diet - Extremely important to follow
+ Smoking with insulin - May increase effects of insulin. Avoid smoking.

RX LABEL PRECAUTIONS:

Take as directed. Follow instructions closely. Avoid alcohol.

***Store all medicines out of childrens reach, away from heat and direct sunlight. Discard old/outdated medications.**
Inform physician(s)/pharmacist of all current medications and any questions that may arise.

See complete prescribing literature for additional information.

CHART 35 : DIGITALIS

EXAMPLES:

CRYSTODIGIN DIGITOXIN DIGOXIN LANOXICAPS LANOXIN

INDICATIONS & EFFECTS:

Arrhythmia, and other cardiac conditions as determined by physician. Effects occur through decreasing sodium and potassium ion transport in cardiac cells, thus increasing inotropic effects (force), refractory period and decreasing conduction rate with resulting improved cardiac output.

DRUG-DISEASE PRECAUTIONS:

Hypo or Hypercalcemia, Hypo or Hyperkalemia, Severe Pulmonary disease, Ventricular fibrillation

DRUG-ALLERGY PRECAUTIONS:

Sensitivity to any ingredients.

PRECAUTIONS:

Hypokalemia - (see side effects below)
Have frequent physician check ups. Take medication the same time each day. DO NOT double dose.

SIDE EFFECTS: Rare to Moderate

REPORT: Hypokalemia (Low Potassium - Muscle cramps, Irregular heartbeat, Breathing problems, Excess thirst or weakness),Hyperkalemia - (Irregular heartbeat, Confusion, Unusual tiredness, Tingling, Breathing problems), Diarrhea, Headache, Loss of appetite, Severe nausea or vomiting, Skin rash, Yellow, Green, White Vision problems, Slow pulse
MONITOR: Tiredness, Upset stomach

*** PREGNANCY/NURSING/AGE/STORAGE/ABUSE PRECAUTIONS:**

Inform physician if pregnant or nursing. Elderly may be more susceptible to effects.

Interacting drugs may be used together in some conditions.

DRUG INTERACTIONS FOR: DIGITALIS
ALL PRODUCTS

+ Alcohol, Amphotericin B, Rifampin - **May seriously** decrease effects of former drug
+ Antacids, Kaolin-pectin, Cholestryramine or Colestepol (if taken at the same time) - **May seriously** decrease effects of former drug
+ Amiodarone, Calcium Channel Blockers, Diuretics Thiazide & Loop, Decongestants, Neuromuscular Blockers, Quinidine, Quinine, Stimulants - **May seriously** increase effects of former drug

DIGOXIN PRODUCTS - In addition

+ Anticholinergics, Antidiabetic Agents, Bronchodilators, Erythromycins, Flecainide, Hydroxychloroquine, Methyldopa, Non steroidal Anti-inflammatories, Propafenone, Prazocin, Spironolactone, Tetracyclines, Trimethoprim - May increase effects of former drug
+ Aminoglycosides, Metoclopramide, Penicillamine, Phenytoin, Procarbazine, Sulfasalazine, Vancomycin - May decrease effects of former drug

DIGITOXIN PRODUCTS - In addition

+ Barbiturates - **May seriously** decrease effects of former drug
+ Tamoxifen - May increase effects of former drug

FOOD/NUTRIENT INTERACTIONS:

+ Food - May decrease rate of absorption

RX LABEL PRECAUTIONS:

Take only as directed. DO NOT double dose.

***Store all medicines out of childrens reach, away from heat and direct sunlight. Discard old/outdated medications.**
Inform physician(s)/pharmacist of all current medications and any questions that may arise.

See complete prescribing literature for additional information.

CHART 36 : DIURETICS POTASSIUM SPARING

EXAMPLES:

ALDACTAZIDE ALDACTONE AMILORIDE DYAZIDE DYRENIUM MAXZIDE MIDAMOR MODURETIC SPIRONOLACTONE + HCTZ SPIRONOLACTONE SPIROZIDE TRIAMTERENE + HCTZ TRIAMTERENE

INDICATIONS & EFFECTS:

Diuretic, Antihypertensive, and other conditions determined by physician. See Chart 37 for the effects of the additional diuretic ingredients in a combination product. Effects of potassium-sparing ingredients occur through decreased reabsorption of sodium, increased potassium conservation and increased excretion of water and decrease in blood pressure. Spironolactone products also inhibit aldosterone.

DRUG-DISEASE PRECAUTIONS:

Acidosis, Hyperkalemia, Kidney or Liver problems, Diabetes, Jaundice, Triomterene in addition, Gout.

DRUG-ALLERGY PRECAUTIONS:

Sensitivity to any ingredients.

PRECAUTIONS:

Dehydration, Increased blood sugar, Sun sensitivity - Use sunscreen outside. Have frequent check ups. Best to avoid alcohol.

SIDE EFFECTS: Rare to Moderate

REPORT: Hyperkalemia (Increased Potassium - Anxiety, Confusion, Slow heartbeat, Numbness, Breathing problems, Weakness), Hyponatremia (Decreased Sodium - Dry mouth, Increased thirst, Tiredness), Back pain, Fever, Severe rash or itching, Unusual bleeding

MONITOR: Nausea, Constipation, Dizziness, Loss of appetite, Decreased libido

*** PREGNANCY/NURSING/AGE/STORAGE/ABUSE PRECAUTIONS:**

Best avoided if pregnant or nursing unless otherwise directed. Elderly may be more sensitive to effects.

Interacting drugs may be used together in some conditions.

DRUG INTERACTIONS FOR: DIURETICS POTASSIUM SPARING

ALL PRODUCTS

+ Ace Inhibitors, Potassium Agents, Cyclosporine - **May seriously** increase side effects of former drug by increasing Potassium level
+ Lithium Digitalis - **May seriously** increase effects of latter drug
+ Non-steroidal Anti-inflammatory Agents, CNS Stimulants, Decongestants - May decrease effects of former drug
+ Antihypertensives - May increase effects of either drug

TRIAMTERENE PRODUCTS - in addition

+ Allopurinol, Colchicine, Probenecid, Sulfinpyrazone - May decrease effectiveness of latter drug with increased uric acid
+ Amatadine - May increase effects of latter drug
+ Diabetic agents, Insulin - May decrease effectiveness of latter with increase blood glucose level

SPIRONOLACTONE PRODUCTS - in addition:

+ Digoxin - May increase effects of latter drug

FOOD/NUTRIENT INTERACTIONS:

+ Excess Potassium Rich Foods i.e. Spinach, Certain types of squash, Whole Baked Potatoe, Watermelon, Salt Substitutes - **May seriously** increase side effects of former drug
+ Diet - Maintain proper diet to maintain electrolyte and nutrition balance

RX LABEL PRECAUTIONS:

Take with food. Unless otherwise directed. Do Not double dose.

***Store all medicines out of childrens reach, away from heat and direct sunlight. Discard old/outdated medications.**
Inform physician(s)/pharmacist of all current medications and any questions that may arise.

See complete prescribing literature for additional information.

CHART 37 : DIURETICS THIAZIDE & LOOP

EXAMPLES:

AQUATENSEN BUMEX BUTMETANIDE CHLORTHALIDONE DIULO DIURIL EDECRIN ENDURON ESIDRIX FUROSEMIDE HYDROCHLOROTHIAZIDE HYDRODIURIL HYGROTON INDAPAMIDE LASIX LOZOL METAHYDRIN NAQUA ORETIC RENESE ZAROXOLYN

INDICATIONS & EFFECTS:

Diuretic, Antihypertensive, and other conditions determined by physician. Effects occur through increased sodium and water excretion, thus reducing extracellular fluid volume, blood pressure, and increasing aldosterone.

DRUG-DISEASE PRECAUTIONS:

Kidney or Liver problems, Diabetes, Nephropathy, Gout, Jaundice, Lupus, Hearing problems with Loop Agents

DRUG-ALLERGY PRECAUTIONS:

Sensitivity to any ingredients. Sulfas, Carbonic Anhydrase Inhibitors, and Diabetic Agents

PRECAUTIONS:

Dehydration, Increased blood sugar, Sun sensitivity - Use sunscreen outside. Have frequent check ups. Best to avoid alcohol.

SIDE EFFECTS: Rare to Moderate

REPORT: Hypokalemia (Low Potassium - Muscle cramps, Weakness, Irregular heartbeat or breathing, Excess thirst), Hyponatremia (Low Sodium - Confusion, Mental changes, Low blood pressure, Irregular heartbeat), Hearing problems, Severe rash or itching, Joint pain, Jaundice, Unusual bleeding

MONITOR: Nausea, Dizziness, Loss of appetite, Decreased libido

*** PREGNANCY/NURSING/AGE/STORAGE/ABUSE PRECAUTIONS:**

Best avoided if pregnant or nursing unless otherwise directed. Elderly may be more sensitive to effects.

Interacting drugs may be used together in some conditions.

DRUG INTERACTIONS FOR: DIURETICS THIAZIDE & LOOP
ALL PRODUCTS

+ Albuterol, Amiodarone, Digitalis, Steroids - **May seriously** increase side effects of latter drug by increased Potassium loss
+ Cholestyramine, Colestipol - **May seriously** decrease effects of former drug
+ Ace Inhibitors, Alcohol, Cyclosporine, Carbonic Anhydrase Inhibitors, Beta Blockers, Lithium - **May seriously** increase side effects of latter drug
+ Methenamine - **May seriously** decrease effectiveness of latter drug
+ Anticoagulants, Antigout Agents, Diabetic Agents, Insulin - May decrease effectiveness of latter drug
+ Non-steroidal Anti-inflammatory Agents, CNS Stimulants, Decongestants - May decrease effects of former drug

LOOP DIURETICS -Bumex, Edecrin, Lasix, In addition

+ Aminoglycosides, Cephalosporines, Quinine - **May seriously** increase side effects of latter drug
+ Probenecid, Phenytoin - **May seriously** decrease effects of former drug

FOOD/NUTRIENT INTERACTIONS:

+ Calcium Supplements (Large amounts) - May increase side effects of latter (Constipation, Nausea, Kidney problems, Confusion, Weakness)
+ Diet - Maintain proper diet to maintain electrolyte and nutrition balance

RX LABEL PRECAUTIONS:

Take with full glass of water. Drink a glass of orange juice daily. Do Not double dose.

***Store all medicines out of childrens reach, away from heat and direct sunlight. Discard old/outdated medications.**
Inform physician(s)/pharmacist of all current medications and any questions that may arise.

See complete prescribing literature for additional information.

CHART 38 : ERGOTAMINE & RELATED DRUGS

EXAMPLES:

BELLERGAL-S CAFERGOT ERGO-CAFF ERGOLOID ERGOMAR ERGONOVINE ERGOSTAT ERGOTAMINE ERGOTRATE HYDERGINE METHERGINE METHYSERGIDE SANSERT WIGRAINE

INDICATIONS & EFFECTS:

Certain types of Headaches, Certain circulation or bleeding problems and other conditions as determined by physician. Effects occur through antagonizing alpha-adrenergic receptors and serotonin.

DRUG-DISEASE PRECAUTIONS:

Heart conditions, Hypo or Hypertension, Eclampsia, Liver or Renal problems, Severe infections

DRUG-ALLERGY PRECAUTIONS:

Sensitivity to any ingredients

PRECAUTIONS:

Avoid alcohol, Smoking, Decreases body temperatures -Use caution in winter, Have frequent check ups. Certain medications require a drug free intervall between courses

SIDE EFFECTS: Moderate

REPORT: Swelling, Chest pain, Anxiety, Confusion, Vision problems, Numbness, Severe headache, Paleness, Irregular Heart rate, Shortness of breath, Blisters

MONITOR: Nausea, Dizziness, Dry mouth

*** PREGNANCY/NURSING/AGE/STORAGE/ABUSE PRECAUTIONS:**

Avoid pregnancy and nursing. Inform physician if pregnant. Elderly may be more sensitive to effects.

Interacting drugs may be used together in some conditions.

DRUG INTERACTIONS FOR: ERGOTAMINE & RELATED DRUGS

+ Beta Blockers, Caffeine, Decongestants, Cocaine, Dopamine, Erythromycins, Troleandomycin, Other Ergot products, Epinephrine or Phenylephrine injection - **May seriously** increase side effects of former drug
+ Oral contraceptives, caffeine, decongestants, Smoking - May increase side effects of former drug
+ Alcohol - May decrease effectiveness of former drug

FOOD/NUTRIENT INTERACTIONS:

+ Excess caffeine, colas, tea - May increase side effects of former drug.

RX LABEL PRECAUTIONS:

Avoid Alcohol and Smoking. Take only as directed. Do Not double dose.

***Store all medicines out of childrens reach, away from heat and direct sunlight. Discard old/outdated medications.**

Inform physician(s)/pharmacist of all current medications and any questions that may arise.

See complete prescribing literature for additional information.

CHART 39 : ERYTHROMYCINS

EXAMPLES:

AZITHROMYCIN BIAXIN CLARITHROMYCIN CLEOCIN CLINDAMYCIN E-MYCIN E.E.S. ERY-TAB ERYC ERYPED ERYTHROMYCIN ERYTHROCIN ILOSONE LINCOCIN PCE ROBIMYCIN TAO TROLEANDOMYCIN WYAMYCIN-S ZITHROMAX

INDICATIONS & EFFECTS:

Antibacterial, Infections and other conditions as determined by physician. Effects occur through bacteriostatic action of binding to ribosomes subunits with resultant decrease in bacteria growth.

DRUG-DISEASE PRECAUTIONS:

Liver problems or hearing problems.

DRUG-ALLERGY PRECAUTIONS:

Sensitivity to any of the ingredients.

PRECAUTIONS:

Jaundice, Adequate fluid intake, Take full course unless otherwise directed

SIDE EFFECTS: Rare

REPORT: Rash, itching, Fever and Sore mouth or throat, Severe stomach pains, Eye or vision problems, Urinary or other skin problems, Unusual tiredness, or Hearing problems
MONITOR: Nausea, Diarrhea, Dizziness, Appetite changes

*** PREGNANCY/NURSING/AGE/STORAGE/ABUSE PRECAUTIONS:**

Inform physician if pregnant or nursing. The estolate form should be avoided if pregnant. Most oral liquid forms should be stored in refrigerator, shaken well and used within specific time period.

Interacting drugs may be used together in some conditions.

DRUG INTERACTIONS FOR: ERYTHROMYCINS

+ Anticoagulants, Alfentanil. Carbamazepine, Cyclosporine, Ergot Alkaloids, Lovastatin, Pravastatin, Simvastatin, Terfenadine, Theophyllines or Xanthines - **May seriously** increase effects of latter drug
+ Digoxin, Disopyramide - May increase effects of latter drug
+ Other Antibiotics, Penicillins, Chloramphenicol, Licomycin - May decrease effectiveness of either drug
+ Contraceptives Oral, Phenytoin - May decrease effects of latter drug

FOOD/NUTRIENT INTERACTIONS:

+ Excess Caffeine (Soda, Tea or Coffee) - May increase effects of latter drug

RX LABEL PRECAUTIONS:

Take with full glass of water. May take with food if upsetting to stomach. Take full course of therapy. Oral Liquids - Shake Well

***Store all medicines out of childrens reach, away from heat and direct sunlight. Discard old/outdated medications.**
Inform physician(s)/pharmacist of all current medications and any questions that may arise.

See complete prescribing literature for additional information.

CHART 40 : ESTROGENS & PROGESTINS

EXAMPLES:

ESTROGENS: CONJUGATED ESTROGEN DIENESTROL DES ESTRACE ESTRADERM ESTRADIOL ESTRATAB ESTROVIS MENEST OGEN PERGONAL PREMARIN TACE. PROGESTINS: AYGESTRIN CYCRIN DEPO-PROVERA NORETHINDRONE NORLUTRATE NORLUTIN MEDROXY-PROGESTERONE PROGESTERONE PROVERA

INDICATIONS & EFFECTS:

Various Estrogen and Progestin deficiencies, Hormone imbalance, Carcinoma, and other conditions as determined by physician. Effects occur through replacement or increased synthesis of nucleuic acids and various proteins involved in replacement.

DRUG-DISEASE PRECAUTIONS:

Breast cancer, Clotting disorders, Hypercalcemia, Abnormal vaginal bleeding, Hepatic disease

DRUG-ALLERGY PRECAUTIONS:

Sensitivity to any ingredients

PRECAUTIONS:

Fluid retention, Smoking - Decreases effectiveness of Estrogens and increases side effects, Read patient package insert carefully, Follow directions closely, Do Not double dose, Notify physician if pregnancy suspected.

SIDE EFFECTS: Rare

REPORT: Breast pain or lumps, Swelling, Menstrual irregularities, Severe headache or pain, Dizziness, Shortness of breath, Vision changes, Numbness

MONITOR: Change in appetite, Acne, Nausea, Cramping, Diarrhea

*** PREGNANCY/NURSING/AGE/STORAGE/ABUSE PRECAUTIONS:**

Avoid if pregnant or nursing, use in young best avoided unless otherwise directed.

Interacting drugs may be used together in some conditions.

DRUG INTERACTIONS FOR:
ESTROGENS
- + Bromocriptine - **May seriously** decrease effects of latter drug
- + Smoking - **May seriously** increase side effects of former drug
- + Steroids, Dantrolene, Cyclosporine - May increase side effects of latter drug
- + Tamoxifen, Thyroid - May decrease effects of latter drug

PROGESTINS
- + Bromocriptine - **May seriously** decrease effects of latter drug

FOOD/NUTRIENT INTERACTIONS:
- + Diet - Maintain balanced diet
- + Megadoses of Vitamin C - May increase side effects of Estrogens

RX LABEL PRECAUTIONS:

Take with food if possible. Do Not double dose. Avoid smoking.

***Store all medicines out of childrens reach, away from heat and direct sunlight. Discard old/outdated medications.**
Inform physician(s)/pharmacist of all current medications and any questions that may arise.

See complete prescribing literature for additional information.

CHART 41 : FLUROQUINOLONES & RELATED DRUGS

EXAMPLES:

CINOBAC CINOXACIN CIPRO CIPROFLOXACIN FLOXIN LOMEFLOXACIN MAXAQUIN NALDIXIC ACID NEGGRAM NORFLOXACIN NOROXIN OFLOXACIN

INDICATIONS & EFFECTS:

Antibiotics used in various infections i.e. Bone or joint, Skin, Urinary, Pulmonary and other conditions as determined by physician. Effects occur through bacterialcidal action on DNA gyrase with resultant decrease in bacterial replication.

DRUG-DISEASE PRECAUTIONS:

Renal or Liver problems and other Central Nervous System disfunctions i.e. history of seizures.

DRUG-ALLERGY PRECAUTIONS:

Sensitivity to any ingredients

PRECAUTIONS:

Possible sun sensitivity - Use sunscreen when outside for extended periods of time, Adequate fluid intake, take with water. Avoid antacids or Sucralfate at the same time. Take two hours apart from Antibiotic.

SIDE EFFECTS: Rare

REPORT: Confusion, Any Urinary problems, Jaundice, Nervousness, Swelling, Joint pain, Vision problems

MONITOR: Diarrhea, Dizziness, Minor itching, Minor upset stomach, Restlessness if taken with caffeine drinks

*** PREGNANCY/NURSING/AGE/STORAGE/ABUSE PRECAUTIONS:**

Best avoided if pregnant or nursing, notify physician. Not recommended in patients under 18 years of age or infants unless otherwise directed.

Interacting drugs may be used together in some conditions.

DRUG INTERACTIONS FOR: FLUROQUINOLONE & RELATED DRUGS
NALDIXIC ACID AND CINOXACIN PRODUCTS

Anticoagulants - **May seriously** increase effects of latter drug

ALL OTHER PRODUCTS

+ Antacids (Aluminum, Calcium and Magnesium), Sucralfate, Ferrous Sulfate - **May seriously** decrease effectiveness of former drug - Take 2 hours after Fluroquinolone.
+ Anticoagulants, Cyclosporine, Theophylline, Xanthines, Caffeine - **May seriously** increase effects of latter drug. (Lomefoxacin less likely to interact)
+ Probenecid - **May seriously** increase effects of former drug
+ Urinary Alkalizers in large amounts i.e. Bicarbonates, Citrates,
+ Carbonic Anhydrase Inhibitors - May decrease solubility of former drug and increase urinary problems

FOOD/NUTRIENT INTERACTIONS:

+ Iron or Zinc - May decrease effect of former. Take two hours after Fluroquinolone.
+ Excess Caffeine (Coffee, Tea, or Colas) - May increase side effects of latter

RX LABEL PRECAUTIONS:

Oral dosages - Take with full glass of water on empty stomach unless otherwise directed. Avoid Antacids at the same time. May cause sun sensitivity - Use sunscreen when outside for extended periods of time.

***Store all medicines out of childrens reach, away from heat and direct sunlight. Discard old/outdated medications.**
Inform physician(s)/pharmacist of all current medications and any questions that may arise.

See complete prescribing literature for additional information.

CHART 42 : FUNGAL AGENTS

EXAMPLES:

ANCOBON DIFLUCAN FLUCYTOSINE FLUCONAZOLE FULVICIN GRIFULVIN GRISEOFULVIN GRIS-PEG GRISACTIN KETOCONAZOLE MYCOSTATIN NILSTAT NIZORAL NYSTATIN

INDICATIONS & EFFECTS:

Antifungals used in various infections i.e. Skin, Urinary, Pulmonary and other conditions as determined by physician. Effects occur through fungistatic action on synthesis of ergosterol, thus damaging cell membrane, or through cell mitosis with resultant decrease in fungal proliferation.

DRUG-DISEASE PRECAUTIONS:

Achlorhydria, Renal or Liver problems, Griseofulvin - in addition, Porphyria and Lupus.

DRUG-ALLERGY PRECAUTIONS:

Sensitivity to any ingredients, Griseofulvin - in addition, possible cross-sensitivity with penicillins.

PRECAUTIONS:

Avoid alcohol, Take full course of therapy, Have frequent checkups. Ketoconazole - in addition, possible eye or skin sun sensitivity - Use sunscreens if outside for extended periods and sunglasses if uncomfortable. Griseofulvin - in addition, may decrease effectiveness of estrogen oral contraceptives - use alternate method during and for one month after therapy.

SIDE EFFECTS: Rare

REPORT: Hepatitis, Dark urine, Stomach pain, Yellow eyes or skin, Loss of appetite, Reddening or blistering of skin, Mouth sores, Fever.

MONITOR: Diarrhea, Dizziness, Minor itching, Minor upset stomach, Sun sensitivity.

*** PREGNANCY/NURSING/AGE/STORAGE/ABUSE PRECAUTIONS:**

Best avoided if pregnant or nursing, notify physician.

Interacting drugs may be used together in some conditions.

DRUG INTERACTIONS FOR: FUNGAL AGENTS

ALL PRODUCTS

+ Alcohol - **May seriously** increase side effects of latter drug

KETOCONAZOLE PRODUCTS - In addition

+ Antacids, Antiulcer H2 blockers, Isoniazid, Rifampin - **May seriously** decrease effects of former drug
+ Anticoagulants, Benzodiazepines, Amiodarone, Anabolics and
+ Androgens, Carbamazepine, Carmustine, Phenytoin, Methotrexate, Nitrofurantoins, Quinidine, Sulfas, Valproic acid - May increase effects of latter drug

FLUCONAZOLE PRODUCTS - In addition

+ Rifampin - **May seriously** decrease effectiveness of former drug+Anticoagulants, Antidiabetic oral agents, Cyclosporine, Phenytoin - **May seriously** increase effects of latter drug

GRISEOFULVIN PRODUCTS - In addition

+ Anticoagulants - **May seriously** decrease effects of lattter drug
+ Barbiturates, Primidone - May decrease effects of latter drug
+ Oral Contraceptives (Estrogen containing) - **May seriously** decrease effectiveness of latter drug with long term griseofulvin therapy. Use alternate or addtional method of contraception during and for one month following therapy.

FOOD/NUTRIENT INTERACTIONS:

+ Food - Take with food if upsetting to stomach

RX LABEL PRECAUTIONS:

Take full course of therapy. Take with full glass of water and with a meal unless otherwise directed. Avoid alcohol.

***Store all medicines out of childrens reach, away from heat and direct sunlight. Discard old/outdated medications.**

Inform physician(s)/pharmacist of all current medications and any questions that may arise.

See complete prescribing literature for additional information.

CHART 43 : GOUT AGENTS

EXAMPLES:

ALLOPURINOL ANTURANE BENEMID COLBENEMID COLCHICINE LOPURIN PROBENECID + COLCHICINE PROBENECID SULFINPYRAZONE ZYLOPRIM

INDICATIONS & EFFECTS:

Gout, Gouty arthritis, Uric Acid, and other conditions determined by your physician. Probenecid is also used to increase effects of certain antibiotics. Other medications may also be used in Gout. Effects occur through changes in uric acid metabolism and decreased accumulation.

DRUG-DISEASE PRECAUTIONS:

Kidney or Liver problems, Ulcer, in addition - Diabetes, High blood pressure with Allopurinol products

DRUG-ALLERGY PRECAUTIONS:

Sensitivity to any ingredients.

PRECAUTIONS:

Have frequent check ups, Avoid alcohol, Follow physicians diet instructions, May cause drowsiness

SIDE EFFECTS: Rare

REPORT: Skin rash, Unusual fever or sore throat, Vision problems, Urinary problems, Numbness, Severe nausea, diarrhea or vomiting

MONITOR: Drowsiness, Tiredness, Loss of appetite, Restlessness

*** PREGNANCY/NURSING/AGE/STORAGE/ABUSE PRECAUTIONS:**

Best avoided if pregnant or nursing. Elderly may be more sensitive to effects.

Interacting drugs may be used together in some conditions.

DRUG INTERACTIONS FOR: GOUT AGENTS

ALL PRODUCTS

+ Alcohol, Antineoplastics, Diuretics Thiazide & Loop, Niacin, Salicylates, Triamterene - May increase Uric Acid or decrease excretion and thus - **May seriously** decrease effectiveness of former drug

ALLOPURINOL PRODUCTS - In addition

+ Alkylating Agents, Azathioprine, Anticoagulants, Captopril, Chlorpropamide, Mercaptopurine, Xanthines, Theophylline, Vidarabine - May increase effects of latter drug

PROBENECID PRODUCTS - In addition

+ Acetaminophen, Acyclovir, Aspirin, Benzodiazepines, Clofibrate, H2 Blockers, Dyphylline, Methotrexate, Salicylates, Non steroidal Anti-inflammatory Agents - May cause **serious** increase in effects of latter drug

SULFINPYRAZONE PRODUCTS - In addition

+ Anticoagulants - May increase effects of latter drug
+ Beta Blockers, Verapamil - May decrease effects of latter drug
+ Aspirin, Salicylates - **May seriously** decrease effects of former drug

FOOD/NUTRIENT INTERACTIONS:

+ High purine diet ie: Anchovies, Bacon, Herring, Liver, Oysters, Sardines, Salmon, Scallops, Trout, Veal, Venison - May cause decrease in effectiveness of former drug. Maintain balanced diet

RX LABEL PRECAUTIONS:

Take with full glass water. May take with food if upsetting to stomach.

***Store all medicines out of childrens reach, away from heat and direct sunlight. Discard old/outdated medications.**
Inform physician(s)/pharmacist of all current medications and any questions that may arise.

See complete prescribing literature for additional information.

CHART 44 : INTERFERONS

EXAMPLES:

ALFERON-N INTERFERON ALFA-N3 INTRON-A INTERFERON ALPHA-2B ROFERON-A INTERFERON ALPHA-2A

INDICATIONS & EFFECTS:

Antiviral, neoplasms, antineoplastic, biological response modifier and other conditions as determined by physician. Effects are through the inhibition of RNA, DNA, cellular proteins and increased phagocytic activity.

DRUG-DISEASE PRECAUTIONS:

Bone Marrow suppression, Renal or Hepatic impairment, Chicken Pox, Certain Herpes, Seizure disorders, Cardiac and Pulmonary disease, Certain DM conditions.

DRUG-ALLERGY PRECAUTIONS:

Sensitivity to any ingredients and egg protein or neomycin with Alpha-N3

PRECAUTIONS:

Vaccines, Infections and minor cuts should be avoided, Must have frequent physician visits to monitor blood tests. Notify any physician seen as to drug and dosage. Use only as directed, do not change brands unless directed. May cause Drowsiness. Avoid Alcohol. Caution if requiring radiation therapy.

SIDE EFFECTS: Moderate

REPORT: Stomach pain, Infections, Fever, Sore Throat, Heart problems, Bleeding problems or blood in urine, Black stools, Confusion, Nervousness, Trouble sleeping, Numbness.

MONITOR: Aching muscles, Chills, Headache, Nausea, Loss of appetite, Itching, Rash, Tiredness, Diarrhea and Loss of Hair.

*** PREGNANCY/NURSING/AGE/STORAGE/ABUSE PRECAUTIONS:**

Best avoided if pregnant and nursing. Elderly may be more sensitive to side effects.

Interacting drugs may be used together in some conditions.

DRUG INTERACTIONS FOR: INTERFERONS

+ Alcohol, Antineoplastics, Antivirals, Narcotics and related agents, Antianxiety agents, Sulfonamides, Procarbazine - **May seriously** increase effects and side effects of former drug

FOOD/NUTRIENT INTERACTIONS:

+ Food - Maintain adequate diet, if nauseated eat lighter portions at one time

RX LABEL PRECAUTIONS:

Avoid alcohol. Use only as directed and Do Not double dose. Have frequent check ups.

***Store all medicines out of childrens reach, away from heat and direct sunlight. Discard old/outdated medications. Inform MD or pharmacist of all current medications and any questions.**

See complete prescribing literature for additional information.

CHART 45 : LITHIUM AGENTS

EXAMPLES:

CIBALITH-S ESKALITH LITHANE LITHIUM LITHOBID LITHONATE

INDICATIONS & EFFECTS:

Tranquilizers, Manic episodes and other conditions determined by physician. Effects occur through the reduction of catecholamine transmitters or cyclic AMP levels.

DRUG-DISEASE PRECAUTIONS:

Sodium depletion, Dehydration, Renal, Heart problems or mental impairment

DRUG-ALLERGY PRECAUTIONS:

Sensitivity to any ingredients.

PRECAUTIONS:

Have frequent check ups, Extreme exercise or sweating, Diuretic Therapy, Drowsiness, Thyroid problems, Decreased Sodium. May require increase in sodium intake.

SIDE EFFECTS: Moderate

REPORT: Diarrhea, Vomiting, Tremors, Severe weakness or drowsiness, Eye or ear problems

MONITOR: Irritability, Confusion, Heart rate, Increased urination, Rash, Thirst

*** PREGNANCY/NURSING/AGE/STORAGE/ABUSE PRECAUTIONS:**

Best avoided if pregnant or nursing unless otherwise directed. Elderly may be more sensitive to effects. Not recommended in children under 12 years of age.

Interacting drugs may be used together in some conditions.

DRUG INTERACTIONS FOR: LITHIUM AGENTS

+ Anticholinergics, Mazindol, Molindone, Non steroidal Anti-inflammatories, Phenytoin, Phenothiazines, Salicylates - **May seriously** increase effects of former drug
+ Ace Inhibitors, Alcohol, Diuretics, Fluoxetine, Methyldopa, Metronidazole, Spectinomycin, Tetracyclines - May increase effects of former drug
+ Antidepressants Tricyclic, Carbamazepine, Haloperidol, Neuromuscular Blockers - May increase effects of either drug Caffeine, Carbonic Anhydrase Inhibitor, Theophyllines, Xanthines - May decrease effects of former drug
+ Iodides (Calcium, Potassium), Iodinated Glycerol, Propylthiouracil, Methimazole - **May seriously** increase effects of latter drug

FOOD/NUTRIENT INTERACTIONS:

+ Low Sodium Diet - **May seriously** increase side effects of former drug. Maintain balanced diet.

RX LABEL PRECAUTIONS:

+ Take with full glass of water and with food. DO NOT double dose.

***Store all medicines out of childrens reach, away from heat and direct sunlight. Discard old/outdated medications.**
Inform physician(s)/pharmacist of all current medications and any questions that may arise.

See complete prescribing literature for additional information.

CHART 46 : MAO INHIBITORS

EXAMPLES:

EUTONYL EUTRON FURAZOLIDONE FUROXONE ISOCARBOXAZID MARPLAN MATULANE NARDIL PARGYLINE PARNATE PHENELZINE PROCARBAZINE TRANYLCYPROMINE

INDICATIONS & EFFECTS:

Antidepressants, Certain blood pressure conditions, and other conditions as determined by physician, Procarbazine - Primarily chemotherapeutic supplement agent. Effects occur primarily through inhibition of monoamine oxidase.

DRUG-DISEASE PRECAUTIONS:

Congestive heart failure, Alcoholism (active), Pheochromocytoma, Renal or Liver problems, Sympathectomy

DRUG-ALLERGY PRECAUTIONS:

Sensitivity to any ingredients

PRECAUTIONS:

Sudden change in blood pressure, Headache, Palpitations, Sun sensitivity - Use sunscreen if prolonged exposure, Certain foods - See interactions, Avoid alcohol, Have frequent check-ups

SIDE EFFECTS: Moderate

REPORT: Headaches, Palpitations, Increased blood pressure, Anxiety, Emotional changes, Dizziness, Weakness, Seizures, Fever, Diarrhea, Chest pain, Nausea

MONITOR: Constipation, Dry mouth, Rash, Weight changes, Edema, Vision, Urinary or Hearing problems

*** PREGNANCY/NURSING/AGE/STORAGE/ABUSE PRECAUTIONS:**

Avoid pregnancy and inform physician if breast feeding. Not recommended in children under 16 years of age unless otherwise directed, Elderly may be much more sensitive to effects.

Interacting drugs may be used together in some conditions.

DRUG INTERACTIONS FOR: MAO INHIBITORS

+ Alcohol, Cocaine, Caffeine, Carbamazepine, Cyclobenzaprine, Rauwolfia, Guanethidine, Methyldopa, Tricyclic Antidepressants, Buspirone, Guanadrel, Levodopa (plain), Reserpine, Decongestants, Antihistimines & Decongestant combinations, OTC Diet aids, CNS Stimulants, L-Tryptophan, Yohimbine - **May seriously** increase effects of former drug - Allow a 7 to 14 day drug free interval before using other drug
+ Fluoxetine - **May seriously** increase effects of either drug - Allow 5 weeks after discontinuing Fluoxetine before using other drug
+ Antidepressants, Tranquilizers, Narcotics, Dextromethorphan - May increase effects of former drug
+ Antidiabetic Agents, Insulin, Antihistimines, Anticoagulants - May increase effects of latter drug

PROCARBAZINE PRODUCTS

+ Methotrexate - **May seriously** increase effects of latter drug, allow 3 days before using methotrexate

FOOD/NUTRIENT INTERACTIONS:

+ Aged cheese: Brie, Camembert, Cheddar, Emmenthaler, Gruyere, Stilton, Meat/fish: Liver, Fermented sausages (Bologna, Pepperoni, Salami, Summer, Shrimp paste), Wines: esp. Chianti, Champagne, Marmite, Excess (Caffeine, Chocolate, or Bananas), Figs, Fava beans, Ginseng, Soy Sauce, Some non-alcoholic & imported beers & ale, Tyramine, L-Tryptophan - **May seriously** increase effects of former drug - Allow 7 to 14 days after therapy before using product

RX LABEL PRECAUTIONS:

May cause drowsiness, Avoid alcohol, Take only as directed, DO NOT double dose

***Store all medicines out of childrens reach, away from heat and direct sunlight. Discard old/outdated medications. Inform physician or pharmacist of all current medications.**

See complete prescribing literature for additional information.

CHART 47 : METHOTREXATE

EXAMPLES:

AMETHOPTERIN FOLEX METHOTREXATE MEXATE MTX RHEUMATREX

INDICATIONS & EFFECTS:

Rheumatoid arthritis, Antineoplastic, Psoriasis and other conditions as determined by physician. Effects are through the inhibition of dihydrofolic acid reductase thus inhibiting cellular replication.

DRUG-DISEASE PRECAUTIONS:

Bone Marrow suppression, Renal or Hepatic impairment, Infection, Urinary problems, Chicken pox, Herpes

DRUG-ALLERGY PRECAUTIONS:

Sensitivity to any ingredients

PRECAUTIONS:

Infections, Dehydration, Joint pain, Vaccines, Must have frequent physician visits to monitor blood tests. Notify any physician seen as to drug and dosage. Take only as directed. Drink plenty of fluids. May cause sun sensitivity - Use sunscreen if outside and as directed.

SIDE EFFECTS: Moderate

REPORT: Diarrhea, Stomach pain, Infections, Fever, Heart problems, Bleeding problems or blood in urine, Black stools, Swelling, Jaundice, Confusion

MONITOR: Hair loss, Nausea, Loss of appetite, Itching Nausea, Rash, Acne

*** PREGNANCY/NURSING/AGE/STORAGE/ABUSE PRECAUTIONS:**

Avoid pregnancy and nursing. Young and elderly may be more sensitive to side effects.

Interacting drugs may be used together in some conditions.

DRUG INTERACTIONS FOR: METHOTREXATE

+ Alcohol, Amiodarone, Cisplatin, Non-steroidal antiinflammatories, Etretinate, Probenecid, Salicylates, Pepto Bismol, Sulfonamides, Procarbazine - **May seriously** increase effects and side effects of former drug
+ Vaccines, Anticoagulants, Thiopurines - **May seriously** increase effects of latter drug
+ Aminoglycosides, Charcoal caps, Folic acid - May decrease effects of former drug

FOOD/NUTRIENT INTERACTIONS:

+ Food - Maintain adequate diet, if nauseated eat lighter portions at one time.
+ Vitamins with Folic Acid - May decrease effects of former drug

RX LABEL PRECAUTIONS:

+ Avoid alcohol and aspirin or salicylates unless otherwise directed. Drink plenty of fluids. Take only as directed and Do Not double dose. Have frequent check ups. Avoid pregnancy.

***Store all medicines out of childrens reach, away from heat and direct sunlight. Discard old/outdated medications. Inform MD or pharmacist of all current medications and any questions.**

See complete prescribing literature for additional information.

CHART 48 : METOCLOPRAMIDE

EXAMPLES:

CLOPRA MAXOLON METOCLOPRAMIDE OCTAMIDE RECLOMIDE REGLAN

INDICATIONS & EFFECTS:

Reflux, Nausea & Vomiting, and other conditions determined by physician. Effects occur through blocking the action of dopamine and thus increasing response of gastrointestinal smooth muscle.

DRUG-DISEASE PRECAUTIONS:

Epilepsy, Gastrointestinal perforation obstruction, Acute asthma, Parkinson's, Renal failure

DRUG-ALLERGY PRECAUTIONS:

Sensitivity to any ingredients or procainamide and procaine

PRECAUTIONS:

Avoid alcohol, May cause restlessness or severe drowsiness especially with other CNS depressant drugs, Do Not double dose.

SIDE EFFECTS: Moderate

REPORT: Sore throat & fever, Severe drowsiness or disorientation, Shortness of breath, Uncontrollable movements, Agitation, Restlessness, Confusion

MONITOR: Drowsiness, Dry mouth, Dizziness, Rash, Constipation, Headache, Weakness, Trouble sleeping

*** PREGNANCY/NURSING/AGE/STORAGE/ABUSE PRECAUTIONS:**

Inform physician if pregnant, may need to avoid nursing, because of effects on child. Elderly and young may be more sensitive to effects. Keep out of reach of children.

Interacting drugs may be used together in some conditions.

DRUG INTERACTIONS FOR: METOCLOPRAMIDE

+ Alcohol, Antidepressants, Barbiturates, Benzodiazepines, Anticonvulsants, Narcotics, Muscle relaxants, Antihypertensives, Sedatives, Antianxiety drugs - **May seriously** increase the side effects of either drug
+ Anticholinergics - **May seriously** decrease the effects of former drug
+ Digoxin, Bromocriptine, Pergolide, - May decrease effects of latter drug
+ Mexiletine - May increase effects of latter drug

FOOD/NUTRIENT INTERACTIONS:

+ Food - Take 30 minutes before meal as directed.

RX LABEL PRECAUTIONS:

May cause drowsiness - Use caution driving & operating machinery.
NEVER Double Dose. Avoid alcohol.

***Store all medicines out of childrens reach, away from heat and direct sunlight. Discard old/outdated medications.**
Inform physician(s)/pharmacist of all current medications and any questions that may arise.

See complete prescribing literature for additional information.

CHART 49 : METRONIDAZOLE

EXAMPLES:

FLAGYL METRONIDAZOLE PROTOSTAT

INDICATIONS & EFFECTS:

Antibacterial and antiprotozoal used in various infections i.e. Skin and soft tissue, Urinary, Pulmonary and other conditions as determined by physician. Effects occur through bacterial-cidal action on DNA thus reducing bacterial proliferation.

DRUG-DISEASE PRECAUTIONS:

Liver problems and other Central Nervous System dysfunctions i.e. history of seizures, Blood dyscrasias

DRUG-ALLERGY PRECAUTIONS:

Sensitivity to any ingredients

PRECAUTIONS:

Avoid alcohol, Dry mouth and metallic taste possible, Treatment for other party if condition was sexually transmitted. Take full course of therapy.

SIDE EFFECTS: Rare to moderate

REPORT: Numbness, Tingling, Swelling, Joint pain, Rash, Fever or sore throat

MONITOR: Diarrhea, Dizziness, Minor itching, Minor upset stomach, Dry mouth, Change in taste, Discoloration of urine

*** PREGNANCY/NURSING/AGE/STORAGE/ABUSE PRECAUTIONS:**

Best avoided if pregnant or nursing, unless otherwise directed, notify physician. Elderly may be more sensitive to effects.

Interacting drugs may be used together in some conditions.

DRUG INTERACTIONS FOR: METRONIDAZOLE

+ Anticoagulants, Alcohol, Disulfuram - **May seriously** increase effects of latter drug
+ Cimetidine - May increase effects of former drug
+ Phenobarbital - May decrease effects of former drug
+ Phenytoin, Carbamazepine, Cisplatin, Cycloserine, Isoniazid, Lithium, Mexiletine, Nitrofurantoin, Quinine, Vincristine - May increase effects of latter drug

FOOD/NUTRIENT INTERACTIONS:

+ Food - May take with meal if upsetting to stomach.

RX LABEL PRECAUTIONS:

+ Avoid alcohol. Take full course of therapy. May discolor urine.

***Store all medicines out of childrens reach, away from heat and direct sunlight. Discard old/outdated medications.**
Inform physician(s)/pharmacist of all current medications and any questions that may arise.

See complete prescribing literature for additional information.

CHART 50 : MUSCLE RELAXANTS SKELETAL

EXAMPLES:

BACOFLEN CARISOPRODOL CHLORZOXAZONE CYCLOBENZAPRINE DANTRIUM DANTROLENE FLEXERIL LIORESAL MAOLATE METHOCARBAMOL NORFLEX NORGESIC ORPHENADRINE PARAFON FORTE D ROBAXIN ROBAXISAL SOMA

INDICATIONS & EFFECTS:

Skeletal muscle relaxant, and other conditions as determined by physician. Effects occur through CNS depressant activity and decreased synaptic activity, with resulting muscle relaxation.

DRUG-DISEASE PRECAUTIONS:

ALL PRODUCTS

Kidney or Liver problems, Mental depression
Orphenadrine - Glaucoma Prostatic problems, Ulcer,
Cyclobenzaprine - Arrhythmias, Hyperthyroidism, Glaucoma

DRUG-ALLERGY PRECAUTIONS: Sensitivity to any ingredients

PRECAUTIONS:

Alcohol and any other CNS depressants, Drowsiness, Unsteadiness, Carisoprodol - Drug dependency history or abuse

SIDE EFFECTS: Moderate

REPORT: Allergic reaction, Confusion, Irregular heartbeat, Severe drowsiness or weakness, Irritability, Nausea or vomiting, Shortness of breath, Vision or Urinary problems
MONITOR: Mild drowsiness, Lightheadedness, Upset stomach, Unusual tiredness, Rash, Discoloration of urine, Dry mouth

*** PREGNANCY/NURSING/AGE/STORAGE/ABUSE PRECAUTIONS:**

Inform physician if pregnant or nursing. Elderly may be more sensitive to effects.

Interacting drugs may be used together in some conditions.

DRUG INTERACTIONS FOR: MUSCLE RELAXANT SKELETAL

ALL PRODUCTS

+ Alcohol, Antianxiety Agents, Barbiturates, Fluoxetine, Other Sedatives or Hypnotics, Narcotics, Tricyclic Ant-depressants - **May seriously** increase side effects of either drug

ORPHENADRINE PRODUCTS - In addition

+ Anticholinergics - May increase side effects of either drug

BACLOFEN PRODUCTS - In addition

+ MAO Inhibitors - May increase effects of either drug
+ Diabetic Agents and Insulin - May decrease effects of latter drug

CYCLOBENZAPRINE PRODUCTS - In addition

+ MAO Inhibitors - **May seriously** increase effects of latter drug (7 to 14 days should elapse between therapies)
+ Tricyclic Antidepressants, Anticholinergics - May increase side effects of latter drug
+ Guanadrel, Guanethidine - May decrease effects of latter drug

FOOD/NUTRIENT INTERACTIONS:

+ Food - Less stomach upset if taken with food

RX LABEL PRECAUTIONS:

May cause drowsiness - Use caution driving and operating machin-ery. Avoid alcohol. DO NOT double dose. May discolor urine.

***Store all medicines out of childrens reach, away from heat and direct sunlight. Discard old/outdated medications.**

Inform physician(s)/pharmacist of all current medications and any questions that may arise.

See complete prescribing literature for additional information.

CHART 51 : NARCOTICS & RELATED DRUGS

EXAMPLES:

CODEINE DARVOCET-N DARVON DEMEROL DILAUDID DOLOPHINE EMPIRIN+COD HYDROCODONE+APAP LOMOTIL LORTAB MEPERIDINE METHADONE MORPHINE MS-CONTIN ORAMORPH PAREGORIC PERCOCET PERCODAN PHENAPHEN+COD PROPOXYPHENE ROXANOL SYNALGOS-DC TALACEN TALWIN TYLENOL+COD TYLOX VICODIN WYGESIC

INDICATIONS & EFFECTS:

Headache, Pain, Diarrhea, Cough and other conditions. Effects occur through CNS depressant activity and possible dependency with long term use.

DRUG-DISEASE PRECAUTIONS:

Alcoholism, Asthma, Breathing or Cardiac problems, Severe diarrhea, Head injury, Kidney or Liver problems, Drug dependency history or abuse, Mental problems; Meperidine, Propoxy-phene - Convulsions.

DRUG-ALLERGY PRECAUTIONS:

Sensitivity to any ingredients

PRECAUTIONS:

Alcohol and any other CNS depressants, Drug dependency history or abuse, Decreased respiration, Drowsiness, Unsteadiness, Possible overdose (Nervousness, Slow heartbeat, Confusion, Dizziness, Low blood pressure, Unconsciousness, Small pupils, Sleeplessness). Possible withdrawal with long term use (Anxiety, Convulsions, Diarrhea, Fast heartbeat, Sweating, Nausea, Cramps, Large pupils)

SIDE EFFECTS: Moderate

REPORT: Note Precautions. Allergic reactions, Breathing problems, Delusions, Irritability, Severe mental depression confusion, drowsiness, Skin discoloration, Unusual weakness or bleeding

MONITOR: Dizziness, Lightheadedness, Nausea, Sleeplessness, Dry mouth, Constipation, Tiredness

*** PREGNANCY/NURSING/AGE/STORAGE/ABUSE PRECAUTIONS:**

Inform physician if pregnant or nursing. Best avoided if pregnant unless otherwise directed by physician. Elderly and children may be more sensitive to effects. May be habit forming.

Interacting drugs may be used together in some conditions.

DRUG INTERACTIONS FOR: NARCOTICS & RELATED DRUGS
ALL PRODUCTS

+ Alcohol, Antidepressants, Anxiety Agents, Anticholinergics, Antihistamines, Barbiturates, Hypnotics, Neuromuscular Blockers, Sedatives - **May seriously** increase side effects of either drug
+ Antihypertensives, Diuretics, Guanethidine, - May increase side effects of latter drug
+ Narcotic Antagonist - **May seriously** increase withdrawal complications in dependent or abusive patient

MEPERIDINE PRODUCTS - In addition

+ Anticoagulants, MAO Inhibitors - **May seriously** increase effects of latter drug

PROPOXYPHENE PRODUCTS - In addition

+ Anticoagulants, Carbamazepine, Doxepin - **May seriously** increase effects of latter drug
+ Nicotine, Smoking - May decrease effects of former drug

MORPHINE PRODUCTS - In addition

+ Zidovudine - **May seriously** increase effects of either drug

METHADONE PRODUCTS - In addition

+ Phenytoin, Rifampin - May decrease effects of former drug

FOOD/NUTRIENT INTERACTIONS:

+ Ascorbic Acid (Vitamin C) - May decrease effects of latter

RX LABEL PRECAUTIONS:

May cause drowsiness - Use caution driving and operating machinery. Avoid alcohol. DO NOT double dose.

***Store all medicines out of childrens reach, away from heat and direct sunlight. Discard old/outdated medications.**
Inform physician(s)/pharmacist of all current medications and any questions that may arise.

See complete prescribing literature for additional information.

CHART 52 : NEOPLASTIC ADDITIONAL AGENTS

EXAMPLES:

ADRIAMYCIN BLENOXANE CERUBIDINE COSMEGEN DTIC EMCYT EULEXIN HEXALEN HYDREA IDAMYCIN LUPRON LYSODREN MATULANE MEGACE MITRACIN MUTAMYCIN NIPENT NOLVADEX NOVATRONE ONCOVIN RUBEX TESLAC VELBAN VELSAR VEPESID VINCASAR ZOLADEX

INDICATIONS & EFFECTS:

Various neoplasms and other conditions as determined by physician. Effects are through: Hormones - counterbalance and interference with cell membrane growth receptor proteins; Antibiotics - inhibits DNA and RNA; Mitotics - cellular inhibition; Hydroxyurea - inhibits RNA; Procarbazine - induces chromosomal breakdown; Mitotane - affects adrenal activity.

DRUG-DISEASE PRECAUTIONS:

Depending on agent - Bone Marrow suppression, Renal or Hepatic impairment, Infection, Cardiac or pulmonary problems.

DRUG-ALLERGY PRECAUTIONS:

Sensitivity to the ingredient

PRECAUTIONS:

Infections, Joint pain, Vaccines, Must have frequent physician visits to monitor blood and urine tests. Notify any physician seen as to drug and dosage. Use only as directed. Drink plenty of fluids.

SIDE EFFECTS: Moderate

REPORT: Infections, Fever, Heart problems, Bleeding problems or blood in urine, Black stools, Swelling, Jaundice, Confusion, Severe drowsiness

MONITOR: Hair loss, Nausea, Loss of appetite, Diarrhea, Hot Flashes with Tamoxifen

*** PREGNANCY/NURSING/AGE/STORAGE/ABUSE PRECAUTIONS:**

Avoid pregnancy and nursing unless otherwise directed.

Interacting drugs may be used together in some conditions.

DRUG INTERACTIONS FOR: NEOPLASTIC ADDITIONAL AGENTS
ALL PRODUCTS
+ Antigout agents - **May seriously** decrease effectiveness of latter drug with increased uric acid
+ Antineoplastics - **May seriously** increase effects of either drug
+ Steroids, Vaccines - May increase risk of infections

ESTRAMUSTINE + Antacids - **May seriously** decrease former drug
TAMOXIFEN + Anticoagulants - **May seriously** increase latter drug
BLEOMYCIN + Digoxin tabs - **May seriously** decrease latter drug
PENTOSTATIN + Allopurinol, FUDR, Vidarabine - **May seriously** increase either drugs effects
DOXORUBICIN + Digoxin - May decrease effects of latter drug
+ Antineoplastics, Cyclophosphamide, Mercaptopurine - **May seriously** increase effects of either drug
+ Barbiturates - **May seriously** decrease effects of former drug

MITOMYCIN + Vincas - May cause **serious** pulmonary reactions
VINCAS + Mitomycin - May cause **serious** pulmonary reactions
+ Digoxin, Phenytoin - May decrease effects of latter drug

ALTRETAMINE + MAO Inhibitors - May cause **serious** hypotension
+ Cimetidine - **May seriously** increase effects of former

PROCARBAZINE + Digoxin - May decreae effects of latter drug
+ Levodopa, Decongestants, OTC diet aids, Stimulants, Tricyclics - **May seriously** increase blood pressure
+ Narcotics - **May seriously** increase effects of latter

MITOTANE + Steriods, Warfarin - **May seriously** decrease latter

FOOD/NUTRIENT INTERACTIONS:

Procarbazine + Tyramine foods (see MAOI's) - May cause **serious** increase in blood pressure
Emcyt + Milk, Calcium - May decrease drugs effect

RX LABEL PRECAUTIONS:

Drink plenty of fluids. Take only as directed. Have frequent check ups. Maintain adequate diet & eat lighter portions more frequently if nauseated.

***Store all medicines out of childrens reach, away from heat and direct sunlight. Discard old/outdated medications. Inform MD or pharmacist of all current medications and any questions.**

See complete prescribing literature for additional information.

CHART 53 : NON-STEROIDAL ANTI-INFLAMMATORIES

EXAMPLES:

ADVIL ANAPROX ANSAID BUTAZOLIDIN CLINORIL DIFLUNISAL DOLOBID FELDENE FENOPROFEN IBUPROFEN INDOCIN INDOMETHACIN KETOPROFEN KETOROLAC LODINE MECLOFENAMATE MECLOMEN MOTRIN NABUN-METONE NALFON NAPROSYN NUPRIN ORUDIS PEDIAPROFEN PHENYLBUTAZONE PIROXICAM PONSTEL RELAFEN RUFEN SULINDAC TOLECTIN TORADOL VOLTAREN

INDICATIONS & EFFECTS:

Arthritis, Pain, Inflammation, Fever, Dysmenorrhea and other conditions as determined by physician. Effects occur through decreased prostaglandin synthesis.

DRUG-DISEASE PRECAUTIONS:

Anemia, Asthma, Nasal Polyps, Certain Cardiac or Blood conditions, Hemophilia, Ulcer, Liver or Renal problems, Lupus

DRUG-ALLERGY PRECAUTIONS:

Sensitivity to any ingredients or severe sensitivity to aspirin (Desensitization may required before use)

PRECAUTIONS:

Avoid DMSO, Have frequent check ups, Avoid Alcohol and Aspirin, Take only as directed, DO NOT Double dose, Surgery. DO NOT take Aspirin while on drug unless otherwise directed. May cause sun sensitivity - use sunscreen if in sun for extended periods. For acute use - may take on empty stomach for short period of time.

SIDE EFFECTS: Rare to Moderate

REPORT: Difficult Breathing, Severe stomach pain, Rash, Itching, Severe drowsiness, Chest pain, Swelling, Increase in blood pressure, Nosebleeds, Confusion, Seizure, Severe headache, Fever, Chills, Sore throat, Cramps, Unusual bleeding, Black stools, Vision problems, Ringing in ears, Urinary problems
MONITOR: Mild fluid retention, Mild drowsiness, Nausea, Flushing, Tiredness, Bloating, Constipation, Diarrhea, Indigestion

*** PREGNANCY/NURSING/AGE/STORAGE/ABUSE PRECAUTIONS:**

Inform physician if pregnant or nursing. Elderly may be more susceptible to effects.

Interacting drugs may be used together in some conditions.

DRUG INTERACTIONS FOR: NON-STEROIDAL ANTI-INFLAMMATORIES

ALL PRODUCTS

+ Alcohol, Anticoagulants, Heparin, Aspirin, Salicylates, Antineoplastics, Lithium, Methotrexate, Moxalactam - **May seriously** increase side effects of latter drug
+ Diuretics, Triamterene - **May seriously** decrease effects of latter drug
+ Probenecid - **May seriously** increase effects of former drug
+ Acetaminophen (long term use), Alcohol, Colchicine, Diabetic Agents, Gold compounds, Insulin, Nifedipine, Penicillamine, Potassium, Rifampin, Steroids (long term use), Sulfinpyrazone, Verapamil - May increase effects of latter drug
  Antacids (at the same time) - May decrease effects of former drug

IBUPROFEN PRODUCTS - In addition

+ Digoxin, Digitalis - May increase effects of latter drug

INDOMETHACIN PRODUCTS - In addition

+ Zidovudine (AZT), Retrovir - **May seriously** increase effects of latter drug
+ Capoten - **May seriously** decrease effects of latter drug

PHENYLBUTAZONE PRODUCTS - In addition

+ Anticonvulsants, Phenytoin, Penicillamine - **May seriously** increase effects of latter drug
+ Methylphenidate, Sulfas - **May seriously** increase effects of former drug

FOOD/NUTRIENT INTERACTIONS:

+ DMSO - May decrease effects of former drug
+ Smoking - May increase stomach distress

RX LABEL PRECAUTIONS:

Take with full glass of water with a meal. Avoid alcohol. May cause drowsiness

***Store all medicines out of childrens reach, away from heat and direct sunlight. Discard old/outdated medications. Inform physician(s) or pharmacist of all current medications and any questions that may arise.**

See complete prescribing literature for additional information.

CHART 54 : ORAL CONTRACEPTIVES

EXAMPLES:

BREVICON DEMULEN ENOVID GENORA LEVLEN LO/OVRAL LOESTRIN MICRONOR MODICON NOR-Q-D NORDETTE NORINYL NORLESTRIN ORTHO-NOVUM OVCON OVRAL OVRETTE TRI-LEVLIN TRI-NORINYL TRIPHASIL

INDICATIONS & EFFECTS:

Pregnancy prevention, Various Estrogen or Progestin deficiencies, Hormone imbalance, and other conditions as determined by physician. Effects occur through hormonal supplementation.

DRUG-DISEASE PRECAUTIONS:

Pregnancy, Breast cancer, Clotting disorders, Hypercalcemia, Abnormal vaginal bleeding, Jaundice

DRUG-ALLERGY PRECAUTIONS:

Sensitivity to any ingredients

PRECAUTIONS:

Take dose at same time each day, Fluid retention, Smoking - May decrease effectiveness of Estrogens and increases side effects, Follow directions closely, Do Not double dose, Have frequent check ups

SIDE EFFECTS: Rare

REPORT: Breast pain or lumps, Swelling, Menstrual irregularities, severe headache or pain, Dizziness, Shortness of breath, Vision changes, Numbness, Abdominal pain, Skin rash, Breakthrough bleeding

MONITOR: Nausea, Cramping, Diarrhea, Tiredness

*** PREGNANCY/NURSING/AGE/STORAGE/ABUSE PRECAUTIONS:**

Avoid if pregnant or nursing. Read patient package insert carefully.

Interacting drugs may be used together in some conditions.

DRUG INTERACTIONS FOR: ORAL CONTRACEPTIVES

+ Barbiturates, Chloramphenicol, Carbamazepine, Ergot, Griseofulvin, Neomycin, Phenytoin, Primidone, Rifampin, Sulfas, Tetracyclines - **May seriously** decrease effectiveness of former drug (Use additional methods to avoid pregnancy)
+ Ampicillin, Penicillin, Metronidazole - May decrease effectiveness of former drug (Use additional methods to avoid pregnancy)
+ Anticoagulants, Bromocriptine, Tamoxifen - **May seriously** decrease effectiveness of latter drug
+ Diabetic Agents, Insulin, Guanethidine, Methyldopa - May decrease effects of latter drug
+ Smoking - **May seriously** increase side effects of former drug
+ Alcohol, Antidepressants Tricyclic, Beta Blockers, Cyclosporine Dantrolene, Maprotiline, Steroids - May increase effects of latter drug

FOOD/NUTRIENT INTERACTIONS:

+ Folic Acid, Pyridoxine - May decrease effects of latter nutrient
+ Mineral Oil - May decrease effectiveness of former drug
+ Vitamin C in large doses (1000 mg/day) - May increase effects of former drug

RX LABEL PRECAUTIONS:

Take with food if possible. Do Not double dose. Avoid smoking. Read package insert closely.

***Store all medicines out of childrens reach, away from heat and direct sunlight. Discard old/outdated medications.**
Inform physician(s)/pharmacist of all current medications and any questions that may arise.

See complete prescribing literature for additional information.

CHART 55 : PENICILLINS

EXAMPLES:

AMOXICILLIN AMOXIL AUGMENTIN BACTOCILL BETAPEN-VK DICLOXACILLIN DYCILL DYNAPEN GEOCILLIN LEDERCILLIN OMNIPEN OXACILLIN PEN-G PEN-VEE-K PENICILLIN VK POLYCILLIN PRINCIPEN PROSTAPHLIN TEGOPEN V-CILLIN-K VEETIDS

INDICATIONS & EFFECTS:

Antibiotics for infections i.e. Upper and lower respiratory tract, Soft tissue, Gastrointestinal, Genitourinary, Skin, Otitis media and other conditions as determined by your physician. Effects occur through bacterialcidal activity on cell wall synthesis or cytoplasm components with resultant decrease in bacterial proliferation.

DRUG-DISEASE PRECAUTIONS:

Bleeding disorders, Gastrointestinal, Mononucleosis and Renal function impairment.

DRUG-ALLERGY PRECAUTIONS:

Sensitivity to Penicillins, Cephalosporin, Penicillamine, Asthma, Eczema, Hay fever, Hives.

PRECAUTIONS:

Avoid alcohol while on therapy, Have frequent check ups, Superinfections, lab test for long term therapy, Diabetics - May cause false urine test results with Copper Sulfite tests.

SIDE EFFECTS: Rare to Moderate

REPORT: Severe diarrhea, Breathing problems, Dizziness, Skin rash, Itching, Cramps, Bloating, Unusual bleeding or blood in urine, Vaginal infections

MONITOR: Mild diarrhea, Nausea, Vomiting, Sore mouth

*** PREGNANCY/NURSING/AGE/STORAGE/ABUSE PRECAUTIONS:**

Inform physician if pregnant/nursing, most liquid preparations require refrigeration - Do Not Freeze, and Shake Well.

Interacting drugs may be used together in some conditions.

DRUG INTERACTIONS FOR: PENICILLINS

+ Other Antibiotics, Heparin, - May increase or decrease effects of either drug
+ Anticoagulants, Aminoglycosides, Cyclosporine, Oral contraceptives (estrogen), Beta Blockers - May decrease effectiveness of latter drug
+ Cholestyramine, Colestipol - **May seriously** decrease effectiveness of former drug if taken at the same time - Take as far apart as possible
+ Methotrexate - May increase side effects of latter drug
+ Probenecid - May increase effects of former drug

INJECTABLE PENICILLINS:

+ Anti-inflammatory Agents, Salicylates, Anturane, ACE inhibitors, Potassium-sparing Diuretics or Potassium products - May increase side effects of latter drug

FOOD/NUTRIENT INTERACTIONS:

PENICILLIN-G

+ Acidic fruit juices - May decrease effectiveness of Penicillin-G if consumed together, take one to two hours apart.

RX LABEL PRECAUTIONS:

Take with full glass of water on empty stomach if possible. Take full course of treatment unless otherwise directed.

***Store all medicines out of childrens reach, away from heat and direct sunlight. Discard old/outdated medications.**
Inform physician(s)/pharmacist of all current medications and any questions that may arise.

See complete prescribing literature for additional information.

CHART 56 : PERIPHERAL VASODILATORS

EXAMPLES:

APRESAZIDE APRESOLINE APRESOLINE-ESIDIX HYDRALAZINE LONITEN MINOXIDIL

INDICATIONS & EFFECTS:

Hypertension and other conditions determined by physician. Effects occur primarily through direct vasodilation of arterioles, thus reducing peripheral resistance and decreased blood pressure.

DRUG-DISEASE PRECAUTIONS:

Cardiac disease, Rheumatic Heart disease, Urinary problems

DRUG-ALLERGY PRECAUTIONS:

Sensitivity to any ingredients.

PRECAUTIONS:

Irregular heartbeat, Dizziness or decrease in alertness, Caution driving, May require tapering dose if physician recommends discontinuing therapy, B-6 requirements may be increased.

SIDE EFFECTS: Moderate

REPORT: Rash, Shortness of breath, Swelling, Urinary problems, Hydralazine Products: Lupus Reaction - (Skin blisters, Chest pain, Discomfort, Joint pain, Sore throat), Minoxidil Products: Irregular heart rate, Excess swelling or weight gain, Chest pain, Excess hair growth, numbness or tingling

MONITOR: Weakness, Nausea, Drowsiness, Diarrhea, Heart rate

*** PREGNANCY/NURSING/AGE/STORAGE/ABUSE PRECAUTIONS:**

Best avoided if pregnant or nursing. Elderly may be more sensitive to effects of medication.

Interacting drugs may be used together in some conditions.

DRUG INTERACTIONS FOR: PERIPHERAL VASODILATORS
ALL PRODUCTS

+ Antihypertensives, other Beta Blockers, Alcohol, Calcium Channel Blockers - May increase effects of either drug
+ Diazoxide - **May Seriously** increase effects of either drug
+ Decongestants, CNS Stimulants, OTC Diet aids, Non steroidal anti-inflammatory agents - May decrease effectiveness of former drug

MINOXIDIL PRODUCTS - In addition

+ Guanethidine, Nitrate Vasodilators - **May seriously** increase effects of either drug

FOOD/NUTRIENT INTERACTIONS:

+ Food - May increase effects of former - Take medication at same time each day
+ Salt - Excessive use may decrease effectiveness of medication
+ Diet - Maintain adequate diet and nutrition, B-6 requirements may be increased

RX LABEL PRECAUTIONS:

Take only as directed. DO NOT double dose. May cause dizziness.

***Store all medicines out of childrens reach, away from heat and direct sunlight. Discard old/outdated medications.**
Inform physician(s)/pharmacist of all current medications and any questions that may arise.

See complete prescribing literature for additional information.

CHART 57 : POTASSIUM PRODUCTS

EXAMPLES:

K-DUR K-LOR K-LYTE K-TABS KAOCHLOR KAON KAY CIEL KLORVESS KLOTRIX MICRO-K POTASSIUM CHLORIDE RUM-K SF TRIKATES TWIN-K

INDICATIONS & EFFECTS:

Hypokalemia (Low Potassium), and other conditions determined by physician. Effects occur through direct replacement of potassium ions.

DRUG-DISEASE PRECAUTIONS:

Acidosis, Addison's disease, Dehydration, Gastrointestinal problems or Ulcer, Hyperkalemia, Infection or Injury, Kidney or Liver problems, Diabetes, Gout, Jaundice, Severe Diarrhea

DRUG-ALLERGY PRECAUTIONS:

Sensitivity to any ingredients.

PRECAUTIONS:

Stomach irritation - Take with food and full glass of water. Mix Powders, Effervescent Tabs and Liquids as directed. Have frequent check ups. Best to avoid alcohol. Follow diet.

SIDE EFFECTS: Rare to Moderate

REPORT: Hyperkalemia (Increased Potassium - Anxiety, Confusion, Slow heartbeat, Numbness, Breathing problems, Weakness), Severe stomach pain, rash or itching, Unusual bleeding, Cramping

MONITOR: Nausea, Diarrhea, Dizziness, Gas

*** PREGNANCY/NURSING/AGE/STORAGE/ABUSE PRECAUTIONS:**

Notify physician if pregnant or nursing. Elderly may be more sensitive to effects.

Interacting drugs may be used together in some conditions.

DRUG INTERACTIONS FOR: POTASSIUM PRODUCTS

+ Ace Inhibitors, Potassium Sparring Diuretics, Cyclosporine - **May seriously** increase side effects of latter drug by increasing Potassium level
+ Digitalis - May increase effects of latter drug
+ Steroids, Corticotropin - May decrease effects of former drug
+ Anticholinergics, Heparin - May increase side effects of former drug

FOOD/NUTRIENT INTERACTIONS:

+ Excess Potassium Foods i.e. Spinach, Certain types of squash, Whole Baked Potato, Watermelon, Salt Substitutes - **May seriously** increase side effects of former drug
+ Diet - Maintain proper diet to maintain electrolyte and nutrition balance

RX LABEL PRECAUTIONS:

Take with food and a full glass of water. Do Not double dose. Mix effervescent Tabs, Liquids and Powders as directed.

***Store all medicines out of childrens reach, away from heat and direct sunlight. Discard old/outdated medications.**
Inform physician(s)/pharmacist of all current medications and any questions that may arise.

See complete prescribing literature for additional information.

CHART 58 : SALICYLATES

EXAMPLES:

A.S.A. ALKA-SELTZER ANACIN ARTHROPAN ASA ASCRIPTIN ASPIRIN CHOLINE SALICYLATE DISALCID EASPRIN EXCEDRIN GEMNISYN MOBIDIN PABALATE SALICYLATE SALSALATE SOD. SALICYLATE TRILISATE ZORPRIN

INDICATIONS & EFFECTS:

Arthritis, Pain, Inflammation, Analgesic, Fever, Dysmenorrhea, Myocardial Infraction Prophylactic. Effects are through prostaglandin synthesis with resultant decreased pain, fever, and inflammation.

DRUG-DISEASE PRECAUTIONS:

Anemia, Asthma, Acute flu or fever in children or teenagers, Gout, Nasal Polyps, Certain Cardiac Bleeding or Blood conditions, Hemophilia, Ulcer, Liver or Renal problems, Lupus

DRUG-ALLERGY PRECAUTIONS:

Sensitivity to any ingredients, Salicylates or severe sensitivity to aspirin, non-steroidal anti-inflammatories (Desensitization may be required before use), tartrazine dye, oil of wintergreen

PRECAUTIONS:

Avoid DMSO, Have frequent check ups, Avoid Alcohol, Surgery. DO NOT take Non-steroidal anti-inflammatories while on drug unless otherwise directed. Do Not take if bottle has strong vinegar odor, May cause false urine sugar test results.

SIDE EFFECTS: Rare to Moderate

REPORT: Ringing in ears, Difficult Breathing, Severe stomach pain, Rash, Itching, Severe drowsiness, Chest pain, Swelling, Increase in blood pressure, Nosebleeds, Confusion, Seizure, Severe headache, Diarrhea, Fever, Chills, Sore throat, Cramps, Unusual bleeding, Black stools, Vision problems, Urinary problems, Uncontrolled flapping, Increased thirst

MONITOR: Mild fluid retention, Mild drowsiness, Nausea, Flushing, Tiredness, Bloating, Constipation, Indigestion, Caffeine containing products may cause stimulation

*** PREGNANCY/NURSING/AGE/STORAGE/ABUSE PRECAUTIONS:**

Inform physician if pregnant or nursing. Elderly may be more susceptible to effects. Children and teenagers may be predisposed to Reye's Syndrome - check with physician before using.

Interacting drugs may be used together in some conditions.

DRUG INTERACTIONS FOR: SALICYLATES

ALL PRODUCTS

+ Anticoagulants, Heparin, Methotrexate, Diabetic Agents & Insulin, Moxalactam, Vancomycin, Thrombolytic Agents, Zidovudine (AZT) - **May seriously** increase effects of latter drug
+ Non-steroidal Anti-inflammatories, Probenecid, Sulfinpyrazone - **May seriously** decrease effects of latter drug
+ Carbonic Anhydrase Inhibitors, Calcium & Magnesium Antacids, Sodium Bicarbonate, Steroids (long term) - May decrease effects of former drug
+ Alcohol, Actaminophen, Phenytoin, Furosemide, Nifedipine, Verapamil - May increase effects of latter drug

BUFFERED CONTAINING PRODUCTS - In addition

+ Ketoconazole, Tetracyclines - **May seriously** decrease effects of latter drug

CAFFEINE CONTAINING PRODUCTS - In addition

+ Lithium - May decrease effects of latter drug
+ MAO Inhibitors, CNS Stimulants - May increase effects of latter drug

FOOD/NUTRIENT INTERACTIONS:

+ Ascorbic Acid, Vitamin K - May decrease latter nutrients levels and supplement mey be required.

RX LABEL PRECAUTIONS:

Take with full glass of water with meal. Avoid alcohol. Take only as directed. Do Not double dose.

***Store all medicines out of childrens reach, away from heat and direct sunlight. Discard old/outdated medications.**
Inform physician(s)/pharmacist of all current medications and any questions that may arise.

See complete prescribing literature for additional information.

CHART 59 : SEDATIVES & HYPNOTICS

EXAMPLES:

CHLORAL HYDRATE DORIDEN EQUANIL ETHCHLORVYNOL MEPROBAMATE MEPROSPAN METHYPRYLON MICRAININ MILTOWN NOCTEC NOLUDAR PLACIDYL VALMID

INDICATIONS & EFFECTS:

Anxiety, Sedative, Hypnotic, Skeletal muscle relaxant, and other conditions as determined by physician. Effects occur through central nervous system depressant activity and possible dependency with long term use.

DRUG-DISEASE PRECAUTIONS:

Alcoholism, Kidney or Liver problems, Mental depression, Breathing problems. Drug dependency history or abuse.

DRUG-ALLERGY PRECAUTIONS:

Sensitivity to any ingredients.

PRECAUTIONS:

Alcohol, other CNS depressants, Drug dependency history or abuse, Possible overdose (Anxiety, Slow heartbeat, Confusion, Dizziness, Low blood pressure, Unconsciousness, Small pupils, Sleeplessness). Possible withdrawal with long term use (Anxiety, Fast heartbeat, Convulsions, Diarrhea, Sweating, Nausea, Cramps, Large pupils)

SIDE EFFECTS: Moderate

REPORT: Confusion, Irregular heartbeat, Severe drowsiness or weakness, Irritability, Restlessness, Nausea or vomiting, Hangover effects, Vision problems

MONITOR: Mild drowsiness, Lightheadedness, Upset stomach, unusual tiredness, Rash

*** PREGNANCY/NURSING/AGE/STORAGE/ABUSE PRECAUTIONS:**

Inform physician if pregnant or nursing. Best avoided if pregnant unless otherwise directed by physician. Elderly and children may be more sensitive to effects. May be habit forming, avoid long term use

Interacting drugs may be used together in some conditions.

DRUG INTERACTIONS FOR: SEDATIVES AND HYPNOTICS
ALL PRODUCTS

+ Alcohol, Antianxiety Agents, Barbiturates, Fluoxetine, Other Sedatives or Hypnotics, Narcotics, Tricyclic Antidepressants - **May seriously** increase side effects of either drug

CHLORAL HYDRATE AND ETHCHLORVYNOL PRODUCTS - In addition

+ Anticoagulants - May increase or decrease effects of latter drug

FOOD/NUTRIENT INTERACTIONS:

Food - Less stomach upset if taken with food

RX LABEL PRECAUTIONS:

May cause drowsiness - Use caution driving and operating machinery. Avoid alcohol. DO NOT double dose. Take with full glass of water. May be habit forming.

***Store all medicines out of childrens reach, away from heat and direct sunlight. Discard old/outdated medications.**
Inform physician(s)/pharmacist of all current medications and any questions that may arise.

See complete prescribing literature for additional information.

CHART 60 : STEROIDS

EXAMPLES:

ARISTOCORT BECONASE CORTISONE DECADRON DELTASONE DEPO-MEDROL DEXAMETHASONE FLORINEF HEXADROL HYDROCORTISONE KENALOG LIQUID PRED MEDROL METHYLPREDNISOLONE NASALIDE ORASONE PEDIAPRED PREDNISONE PREDNISOLONE TRIAMCINOLONE VANCERIL

INDICATIONS & EFFECTS:

Adrenal or Allergic Conditions, Asthma, Inflammation, Rhinitis, Immunosuppressant, & other conditions as determined by physician. Effects occur through replacement or synthesis of steroids.

DRUG-DISEASE WARNINGS (Primarily Oral/Injectable Dosage Forms):

Vaccines, AIDS, Certain infections (fungal, bacterial, viral), Diabetes, Certain cardiac conditions, Active ulcer, Myasthenia gravis, TB

DRUG-ALLERGY PRECAUTIONS:

Sensitivity to any ingredients

PRECAUTIONS:

May increase blood sugar, Skin tests, Vaccines, Surgery, Have frequent check-ups, May need to decrease dosage gradually before discontinuing - follow physician instructions closely

SIDE EFFECTS: Moderate

REPORT: Vision problems, Swelling, Acne, Rash, Irregular heartbeat, Flu, Muscle weakness or cramps, Severe nausea, Confusion, Restlessness, Mood changes, Depression, Increased thirst or frequent urination, Bleeding problems

MONITOR: Headache, Sweating, Flushing, Dizziness, Indigestion, Cough, Water retention, Increased appetite

* **PREGNANCY/NURSING/AGE/STORAGE/ABUSE PRECAUTIONS:**

Inform physician if pregnant or nursing. May suppress growth in children.

Interacting drugs may be used together in some conditions.

DRUG INTERACTIONS FOR: STEROIDS

ALL PRODUCTS (Oral tablets & Injectables more likely to Interact than inhalation products)

- + Antacids (at the same time), Rifampin - **May seriously** decrease effects of former drug
- + Diabetic Agents, Insulin, Diuretics (Potassium Sparing), Potassium products, Somatropin - **May seriously** decrease effects of latter drug
- + Digitalis, Diuretics (Thiazide & Loop), Amphotericin B, Carbonic Anhydrase Inhibitors, Vaccines - **May seriously** increase effects of latter drug
- + Ritodrine - **May seriously** increase effects of former drug
- + Alcohol, Non-steroidal Anti-inflammatories, Anabolics, Anticholinergics, Anti-depressants Tricyclic - May increase side effects of latter drug
- + Anticoagulants, Isoniazid, Mexiletine, Salicylates - May decrease effects of latter drug
- + Oral contraceptives - May increase effects of former drug

DEXAMETHASONE PRODUCTS - In addition

- + Aminoglutethimide, Ephedrine - **May seriously** decrease effects of former drug

METHYLPREDNISOLONE PRODUCTS - In addition

- + Erythromycins, Ketoconazole - **May seriously** increase effects of former drug

FOOD/NUTRIENT INTERACTIONS:

Diet - May require increased Folic Acid, protein, & potassium and decreased sodium with long term use.

RX LABEL PRECAUTIONS:

Take with food. Avoid alcohol. Do Not double dose.

***Store all medicines out of childrens reach, away from heat and direct sunlight. Discard old/outdated medications.**

Inform physician(s)/pharmacist of all current medications and any questions that may arise.

See complete prescribing literature for additional information.

CHART 61 : SULFA & RELATED COMBINATIONS

EXAMPLES:

AZO-GANTANOL AZO-GANTRISIN AZULFIDINE BACTRIM EES/SULF GANTANOL GANTRISIN PEDIAZOLE PROLOPRIM RENOQUID SEPTRA SMZ/TMP SULFAMETHOXAZOLE SULFASALAZINE SULFATRIM TRIMETHOPRIM TRIMPEX TRIPLE SULFA UROPLUS

INDICATIONS & EFFECTS:

Antibacterial, Infections and other conditions as determined by physician. Effects occur primarily through bacteriostatic activity on enzymes incorporating PABA in dihydrofolic acid with resultant decrease in bacterial proliferation.

DRUG-DISEASE PRECAUTIONS:

Megaloblastic Anemia, G6 PD deficiency, Liver or Urinary problems, Blood dyscrasias, Porphyria

DRUG-ALLERGY PRECAUTIONS:

Sensitivity to Diabetic Agents or Diuretics, Carbonic Anhydrase Inhibitors, Sulfas and any ingredients

PRECAUTIONS:

Sun sensitivity - Use sunscreen when outside for extended periods, Maintain Adequate fluid intake, Take full course of therapy unless otherwise directed

SIDE EFFECTS: Rare to Moderate

REPORT: Rash, itching, Fever and Sore throat, Aches and Pains, Eye or vision problems, Urinary or other skin problems Unusual tiredness, Difficult breathing

MONITOR: Nausea, Diarrhea, Dizziness, Appetite changes

*** PREGNANCY/NURSING/AGE/STORAGE/ABUSE PRECAUTIONS:**

Avoid in pregnancy and breast feeding - Not recommended in infants less than 2 months old. Elderly may be more sensitive to effects especially if on diuretic therapy. Sulfacytine (Renoquid) not recommended in patients under 14 years old.

Interacting drugs may be used together in some conditions.

DRUG INTERACTIONS FOR: SULFA & RELATED COMBINATIONS
ALL PRODUCTS

+ Methotrexate, Mercaptopurine - **May seriously** increase effects of latter drug
+ Oral Contraceptives - May decrease effects of latter with long term use of former drug

SULFA PRODUCTS - In addition

+ Anticoagulants, Diabetic Agents, Methenamine, Phenytoin - **May seriously** increase effects of latter drug
  Probenecid, Sulfinpyrazone - **May seriously** increase side effects of former drug
+ Digoxin, Penicillins, Vitamin K - May decrease effects of latter drug

TRIMETHOPRIM PRODUCTS - In addition

+ Cyclosporine, Dapsone, Procainamide - **May seriously** increase effects of latter drug
+ Rifampin - **May seriously** increase effects of former drug

FOOD/NUTRIENT INTERACTIONS:

+ Water - May decrease side effects of former drug. Take with full glass of water.

RX LABEL PRECAUTIONS:

Take with full glass of water. May take with food. Use sunscreen outside. Take full course of therapy. Oral Liquids - Shake Well

***Store all medicines out of childrens reach, away from heat and direct sunlight. Discard old/outdated medications.**
Inform physician(s)/pharmacist of all current medications and any questions that may arise.

See complete prescribing literature for additional information.

CHART 62 : TETRACYCLINES

EXAMPLES:

ACHROMYCIN-V DECLOMYCIN DORYX DOXYCYCLINE MINOCIN MINOCYCLINE MONODOX OXYTETRACYCLINE PANMYCIN ROBITET RONDOMYCIN SUMYCIN TERRAMYCIN TETRACYCLINE VIBRAMYCIN VIBRATAB

INDICATIONS & EFFECTS:

Antibiotics for infections i.e. Acne, Respiratory tract, Soft tissue, Gastrointestinal, Genitourinary, Skin, Otitis media and other conditions as determined by your physician. Bacteriostatic effects occur through blocking protein synthesis at the ribosome complex thus inhibiting bacterial replecation.

DRUG-DISEASE PRECAUTIONS:

Renal function impairment or Liver problems.

DRUG-ALLERGY PRECAUTIONS:

Sensitivity to Tetracyclines. Lidocaine or Procaine sensitivity for injectable forms of Tetracyclines.

PRECAUTIONS:

Sun sensitivity - Use sunscreen when outside for extended periods, Best to avoid alcohol while on therapy, Have frequent check ups, Antacids, Calcium, Iron or Magnesium Supplements and Dairy products should not be taken at the same time, Take two hours after.

SIDE EFFECTS: Rare to Moderate

REPORT: Severe diarrhea, Increased urination, Skin rash, Thirst, Unusual tiredness, Vaginal infections

MONITOR: Dizziness, Mild diarrhea, Nausea, Vomiting, Sore mouth

*** PREGNANCY/NURSING/AGE/STORAGE/ABUSE PRECAUTIONS:**

Best avoided if pregnant or nursing unless otherwise directed. Avoid in children less than 8 years old. Do Not take outdated Tetracyclines.

Interacting drugs may be used together in some conditions.

DRUG INTERACTIONS FOR: TETRACYCLINES

ALL PRODUCTS

+ Antacids, Bismuth Subsalicylate, Quinapril,Calcium, Magnesium, Iron and Zinc Supplements - **May seriously** decrease effectiveness of former drug. Take two hours apart
+ Oral contraceptive (long term use of both), Penicillin, Heparin - May decrease effects of latter drug
+ Anticoagulants, Digoxin, Lithium, Theophylline (long term use of both) - May increase effects of latter drug

DOXYCYCLINE PRODUCTS: In addition

+ Barbiturates, Carbamazepines, Phenytoin, Rifampin - May decrease effectiveness of former drug

FOOD/NUTRIENT INTERACTIONS:

+ Calcium and Iron Supplements, Vitamins with Zinc, Milk or dairy products - **May seriously** decrease effectiveness of former. Take two hours after Tetracycline dose as directed.
+ Diet - Long term Tetracycline use may decrease multi vitamins and minerals, a daily supplement taken 2 hours after Tetracycline may be advisable.

RX LABEL PRECAUTIONS:

Take with full glass of water on empty stomach if possible. Take full course of treatment unless otherwise directed. Use sunscreen if outside.

***Store all medicines out of childrens reach, away from heat and direct sunlight. Discard old/outdated medications.**
Inform physician(s)/pharmacist of all current medications and any questions that may arise.

See complete prescribing literature for addltlonal information.

CHART 63 : THEOPHYLLINES & XANTHINES

EXAMPLES:

AMINOPHYLLINE AMINOPHYLLINE CAFFEINE CHOLEDYL DILOR DYPHYLLINE ELIXOPHYLLIN LABID LUFYLLIN MARAX NODOZ QUIBRON RESPBID SLO-BID SLO-PHYLLIN SOMOPHYLLIN SUSTAIRE T-PHYL TEDRAL THEO-24 THEO-DUR THEOBID THEOLAIR THEON THEOVENT-LA UNIPHYL

INDICATIONS & EFFECTS:

Asthma, Bronchitis, Emphysema and other conditions as determined by physician. Effects occur through relaxation of bronchial smooth muscle with resultant decreased airway resistance. Caffeine effects are primarily through CNS stimulation.

DRUG-DISEASE PRECAUTIONS:

Arrhythmias, Congestive heart failure, Active ulcer, Certain liver or Renal problems.

DRUG-ALLERGY PRECAUTIONS:

Sensitivity to any ingredients or Aminophylline.

PRECAUTIONS:

Report Flu, fever or diarrhea; have frequent check-ups. Watch caffeine intake; avoid alcohol.

SIDE EFFECTS: Rare to Moderate

REPORT: Irregular heartbeat or breathing, Seizures, Heartburn, Confusion, Diarrhea, Flushing, Restlessness, Twitching, Severe headache, Frequent urination, Cramps, Weakness, Vomiting
MONITOR: Skin rash, Nausea, Nervousness

*** PREGNANCY/NURSING/AGE/STORAGE/ABUSE PRECAUTIONS:**

Best avoided if pregnant or nursing unless otherwise directed by physician. Children and elderly may be more susceptible to effects.

Interacting drugs may be used together in some conditions.

DRUG INTERACTIONS FOR: THEOPHYLLINES & XANTHINES
ALL PRODUCTS

+ Erythromycins, Troleandomycin, Ciprofloxin, Cimetidine, Ranitidine, Nicotine gum/patch, Beta Blockers - **May seriously** increase effects of former drug
+ Phenytoin, Smoking - **May seriously** decrease effects of former drug
+ Interferon alpha-2a, Temafloxacin, Lomefoxacin, Tetracyclines (long term), Allopurinol, Anesthetics, Calcium Channel blockers, Flu vaccine, Mexiletine,Thiabendazole - May increase effects of former drug
+ Bronkodilators, CNS stimulants, Decongestants, Diet aids, Carbamazepine, Phenobarbital, Primidone, Rifampin - May decrease effects of former drug
+ Lithium, Oral estrogen contraceptives - May decrease effectiveness of latter drug

DYPHYLLINE PRODUCTS - in addition

+ Probenecid - **May seriously** increase effects of former drug

FOOD/NUTRIENT INTERACTIONS:

+ Smoking, High diet of charcoal broiled foods - **May seriously** decrease effects of former drug
+ Food (at the same time), Caffeine (large amounts)- **May seriously** increase effects of former drug
+ High protein diet - May decrease effects of former drug
+ Low protein diet - May increase effects of former drug

RX LABEL PRECAUTIONS:

Take on an empty stomach with water unless otherwise directed. Take only as directed. Do Not miss or double dose.

***Store all medicines out of childrens reach, away from heat and direct sunlight. Discard old/outdated medications.**
Inform physician(s)/pharmacist of all current medications and any questions that may arise.

See complete prescribing literature for additional information.

CHART 64 : THYROIDS

EXAMPLES:

ARMOUR THYROID CYTOMEL EUTHROID L-THYROXINE LEVOTHROID LEVOTHYROXINE LIOTHYRONINE LIOTRIX PROLOID SYNTHROID THYRAR THYROGLOBULIN THYROID THYROLAR

INDICATIONS & EFFECTS:

Various Thyroid diseases, and other conditions as determined by physician. Effects occur through thyroid replacement and metabolism.

DRUG-DISEASE PRECAUTIONS:

Adrenal problems, Diabetes, Certain Heart or Vascular Disease, High blood pressure

DRUG-ALLERGY PRECAUTIONS:

Sensitivity to any ingredients

PRECAUTIONS:

Diarrhea may decrease absorption, Overexertion, Surgery; Should not be used in diet plan unless diagnosed with Hypothyroidism

SIDE EFFECTS: Rare

REPORT: Rash, Excess Thyroid, Severe headache or fever, Fast or irregular heartbeat, Shortness of breath, Nervousness, Cramps, Sweating, Diarrhea, Sleeplessness

MONITOR: Constipation, Weakness, Weight gain

*** PREGNANCY/NURSING/AGE/STORAGE/ABUSE PRECAUTIONS:**

Inform physician if pregnant or nursing. Elderly and young may require lower dosages.

Interacting drugs may be used together in some conditions.

DRUG INTERACTIONS FOR: THYROIDS

+ Anticoagulants, CNS Stimulants, Decongestants - **May seriously** increase effects of latter drug
+ Cholestyramine, Colestipol - **May seriously** decrease effects of former drug (Take four hours apart)
+ Beta Blockers, Estrogens, Lovastatin, Excess Iodine or Iodide - May decrease effects of former drug
+ Amiodarone - May decrease effects of former drug (Liothyronine may not be affected)
+ Diabetic Agents and Insulin, Steroids - May decrease effects of latter drug
+ Maprotiline - May increase effects of former drug

FOOD/NUTRIENT INTERACTIONS:

Diet - Maintain balanced diet

RX LABEL PRECAUTIONS:

Take on empty stomach if possible. Do Not double dose

***Store all medicines out of childrens reach, away from heat and direct sunlight. Discard old/outdated medications.**
Inform physician(s)/pharmacist of all current medications and any questions that may arise.

See complete prescribing literature for additional information.

CHART 65 : TRANQUILIZERS

EXAMPLES:

CHLORPROMAZINE CLOZAPINE CLOZARIL COMPAZINE FLUPHENAZINE HALDOL HALOPERIDOL LOXAPINE LOXITANE MELLARIL MESORIDAZINE MOBAN NAVANE PERMITIL PERPHENAZINE PROCHLORPERAZINE PROLIXIN PROMAZINE SERENTIL SPARINE STELAZINE TARACTAN THIORIDAZINE THIOTHIXENE THORAZINE TRIFLU-PERAZINE TRILAFON

INDICATIONS & EFFECTS:

Nervousness, Psychosis, Behavior or Emotional conditions and other conditions as determined by physician. Effects occur primarily through antagonizing dopaminergic binding.

DRUG-DISEASE PRECAUTIONS:

Active alcoholism, Severe depression, Cardiovascular disease, Seizures, Liver or renal problems: Haloperidol - in Parkinson's: Clozapine - Blood disorders: Phenothiazines - in Reye's Syndrome

DRUG-ALLERGY PRECAUTIONS:

Sensitivity to any ingredients, Prior allergic reactions

PRECAUTIONS:

Uncontrolled movements, Avoid Alcohol, Possible heat stroke, Surgery, Sun sensitivity - use sun screen if extended exposure to the sun, Avoid tanning salons, Have frequent check-ups

SIDE EFFECTS: Rare to Moderate

REPORT: Irregular movements or heart rate, Increase or decrease in blood pressure, Dizziness, Fever, Chills, Sore throat, Anxiety, Confusion, Severe headache, Unusual bleeding, Hearing, Abdominal, Urinary or breathing problems, Seizures, Rash, Hot dry skin

MONITOR: Drowsiness, Constipation, Nausea, Increased or decreased sweating, Dry mouth, Weight gain, Stiffness

*** PREGNANCY/NURSING/AGE/STORAGE/ABUSE PRECAUTIONS:**

Avoid pregnancy and nursing, some are not recommended in children, elderly may be much more susceptible to effects.

Interacting drugs may be used together in some conditions.

DRUG INTERACTIONS FOR: TRANQUILIZERS

ALL PRODUCTS

- \+ Alcohol, Amantadine, Antidepressants, Anticonvulsants, Anti anxiety Agents, Antihistamines, Anticholinergics, Barbiturates, Muscle relaxants, Narcotics, Sedatives - **May seriously** increase effects of latter drug

PHENOTHIAZINES PRODUCTS - In addition

- \+ Lithium - **May seriously** decrease effects of former drug
- \+ Beta Blockers - May increase effects of either drug
- \+ Levodopa, Epinephrine - **May seriously** decrease effects of latter drug

HALOPERIDOL PRODUCTS - In addition

- \+ Lithium, Methyldopa - **May seriously** increase effects of former drug
- \+ Levodopa, Epinephrine - **May seriously** decrease effects of latter drug

THIOTHIXENE PRODUCTS - In addition

- \+ Quinidine - **May seriously** increase effects of latter drug
- \+ Levodopa, Epinephrine - **May seriously** decrease effects of latter drug

MOLINDONE PRODUCTS - In addition

- \+ Lithium - **May seriously** increase effects of former drug
- \+ Insulin, Diabetic Agents - **May seriously** decrease effects of latter drug
- \+ Beta Blockers - **May seriously** increase effects of latter drug

CLOZAPINE PRODUCTS - In addition

- \+ Lithium - **May seriously** increase effects of former drug
- \+ Antineoplastics - **May seriously** increase effects of latter drug

FOOD/NUTRIENT INTERACTIONS:

Clozapine Products + smoking - May decrease effectiveness of former drug

RX LABEL PRECAUTIONS:

Avoid alcohol, May take with food, May cause drowsiness. Take only as directed. DO NOT double dose.

***Store all medicines out of childrens reach, away from heat and direct sunlight. Discard old/outdated medications. Inform physician(s) or pharmacist of all current medications and any questions that may arise.**

See complete prescribing literature for additional information.

CHART 66 : URINARY ANTISEPTICS

EXAMPLES:

ATROSEPT FURADANTIN HIPREX MACROBID MACRODANTIN MANDELAMINE METHENAMINE NITROFURANTOIN PROSED/DS UREX URISED URITIN

INDICATIONS & EFFECTS:

Antibiotics used in various infections primarily urinary tract and other conditions as determined by physician. Effects occur through bacterialcidal action with formaldehyde formation in acidic urinary pH with methenamine and by altering bacterial ribosomes with nitrofurantoins.

DRUG-DISEASE PRECAUTIONS:

Renal or Liver problems for all products. G6PdD deficiency, neuropathy and pulmonary disease in addition with nitrofurantoins.

DRUG-ALLERGY PRECAUTIONS:

Sensitivity to any ingredients.

PRECAUTIONS:

Adequate fluid intake, take with a full glass of water and with food. Methenamine - Avoid citrus fruits, milk and dairy products, use cranberry juice to lower urine pH. Nitrofurantoins - False positive urine glucose test with copper sulfate. Have frequent check-ups even with long term therapy.

SIDE EFFECTS: Rare

REPORT: Pneumonitis, Chest pain, Chills, Fever, Cough, Breathing Problems, Weakness, Rash, Headache, Any urinary problems, Jaundice, Nervousness, Swelling, Numbness or tingling.

MONITOR: Diarrhea, Dizziness, Minor itching, Minor upset stomach.

*** PREGNANCY/NURSING/AGE/STORAGE/ABUSE PRECAUTIONS:**

Best avoided if pregnant or nursing, notify physician. Not recommended in young or infants unless otherwise directed.

Interacting drugs may be used together in some conditions.

DRUG INTERACTIONS FOR: URINARY ANTISEPTICS
NITROFURANTOIN PRODUCTS

+ Antacids, Nalidixic acid - May decrease effects of former drug. Antacids may be taken 2 hours after former drug
+ Alcohol, Probenecid, Sulfinpyrazone - **May seriously** increase side effects of former drug.
+ Antidiabetic oral agents, Carbamazepine, Chloramphenicol, Cisplatin, Cyclosporine, DPT, Ethambutol, Isoniazid, Methydopa, Metronidazole, Mexiletine, Other antibiotics, Procainamide, Quinidine, Quinine, Sulfas - May increase side effects of either drug

METHENAMINE PRODUCTS

+ Thiazide Diuretics - **May seriously** decrease effects of former drug
+ Sulfamethiazole, Urinary Alkalizers in large amounts i.e. Bicarbonates, Citrates, Carbonic Anhydrase Inhibitors - May decrease solubility of former drug effectiveness and increase urinary problems

FOOD/NUTRIENT INTERACTIONS:
METHENAMINE PRODUCTS

+ Citrus fruits and juices - May decrease effects of former drug, use cranberry juice.

RX LABEL PRECAUTIONS:

Take with full glass of water and with food unless otherwise directed. May discolor urine.

***Store all medicines out of childrens reach, away from heat and direct sunlight. Discard old/outdated medications.**
Inform physician(s)/pharmacist of all current medications and any questions that may arise.

See complete prescribing literature for additional information.

CHART 67 : VASODILATORS

EXAMPLES:

ARLIDIN CARDILATE CERESPAN CYCLANDELATE CYCLOSPASMOL DEPONIT DILATRATE-SR DIPYRIDAMOLE ISMO ISORDIL ISOSORBIDE ISOXSURPINE MINITRAN NITRODUR NITROGARD NITROGLYCERIN NITROL NITROLINGUAL NITROSTAT PAPAVERINE PAVABID PERITRATE PERSANTINE SORBITRATE VASODILAN

INDICATIONS & EFFECTS:

Angina, Hypertension, Certain heart conditions, and other conditions as determined by physician. Effects occur primarily through arterial dilation and reduced myocardial oxygen demand.

DRUG-DISEASE PRECAUTIONS:

Head trauma, Severe anemia, Glaucoma, Hyperthyroidism, Various cardiac conditions

DRUG-ALLERGY PRECAUTIONS:

Sensitivity to any ingredients, Nitrates or Nitrites

PRECAUTIONS:

Avoid Alcohol. Have regular blood pressure determinations and heart rate checks

SIDE EFFECTS: Rare

REPORT: Blurred vision, Severe headache, Skin rash or discoloration of skin or lips, Dry mouth, Dizziness, Irregular heartbeat, Shortness of breath, Weakness, Fever or convulsions.
MONITOR: Heart rate, Flushing, Nausea, Lightheadedness, Restlessness, Low blood pressure

*** PREGNANCY/NURSING/AGE/STORAGE/ABUSE PRECAUTIONS:**

Inform physician if pregnant or nursing. Elderly may be more susceptible to effects.

Interacting drugs may be used together in some conditions.

DRUG INTERACTIONS FOR: VASODILATORS

+ Alcohol, Antihypertensives, Calcium channel blockers & other Vasodilators - **May seriously** increase effects of latter drug
+ Narcotic analgesics, Tranquilizers, Diuretics - May increase effects of latter drug
+ CNS Stimulants, Decongestants, OTC diet aids - May decrease effects of former drug

FOOD/NUTRIENT INTERACTIONS:
SUBLINGUAL PRODUCTS

Smoking - May decrease effects of former drug.

RX LABEL PRECAUTIONS:

Avoid alcohol, use only as directed, Do Not double dose. Read patient instructions carefully.

***Store all medicines out of childrens reach, away from heat and direct sunlight. Discard old/outdated medications.**
Inform physician(s)/pharmacist of all current medications and any questions that may arise.

See complete prescribing literature for additional information.

CHART 68 : VIRAL AGENTS

EXAMPLES:

ACYCLOVIR AZIDOTHYMIDINE AZT DDC DDI DIDEOXY-CYTIDINE DIDEOXYINOSINE RETROVIR VIDEX ZIDOVU-DINE ZOVIRAX

INDICATIONS & EFFECTS:

Acyclovir, Zovirax - Herpes, Chickenpox
Dideoxynucleosides - AZT, Retrovir, Zidovudine, Videx, Dideoxyinosine, DDI, Acquired Immunodeficiency Syndrome
Viralstatic effects occur primarily through inhibiting DNA replication.

DRUG-DISEASE PRECAUTIONS:

Acyclovir - Dehydration, Renal problems
Dideoxynucleosides - Bone marrow depression, Hepatic problems, Folic acid or B12 deficiency

DRUG-ALLERGY PRECAUTIONS:

Sensitivity to any ingredients.

PRECAUTIONS:

Avoid sexual contact or use a condom; obtain frequent check-ups and blood tests. Take only as directed.

SIDE EFFECTS: Moderate

REPORT: Acyclovir - Abdominal pain, urinary problems, nausea, vomiting, unusual tiredness. Dideoxynucleosides - Anemia, fever, chills, sore throat, abdominal pain, confusion, vision problems, seizure, pale skin.

MONITOR: Headache, mild nausea, insomnia.

***PREGNANCY NURSING AGE STORAGE ABUSE PRECAUTIONS:**

Best avoided if pregnant or nursing, elderly may be more susceptible to effects.

Interacting drugs may be used together in some conditions.

DRUG INTERACTIONS FOR: VIRAL AGENTS

ACYCLOVIR PRODUCTS:

+ Probenecid - **May seriously** increase side effects of former drug
+ Interferon or Methotrexate injection - May increase effects of latter drug
+ Aminoglycosides, Cyclosporine, Lithium, Methotrexate, Neomycin, Polymixins, Sulfonamides, Vancomycin - With IV Acyclovir - **May seriously** increase side effects of latter drug

DIDEOXYNUCLEOSIDES PRODUCTS:

+ Probenecid, Ganciclovir - **May seriously** increase effects of former drug
+ Acetaminophen, Aspirin, Benzodiazepines, Cimetidine, Indomethacin, Sulfonamides - May increase effects of former drug
+ Amphotercin B, Antineoplastics, Hydroxyurea, Interferon - May increase effects of either drug
+ Acyclovir - May cause severe drowsiness

FOOD/NUTRIENT INTERACTIONS:

+ Dideoxynucleosides may increase Folic acid or B-12 deficiencies and supplementation may be required.

RX LABEL PRECAUTIONS:

Take with food. Use only as directed. DO NOT double dose.

***Store all medicines out of childrens reach, away from heat and direct sunlight. Discard old/outdated medications.**

Inform physician(s)/pharmacist of all current medications and any questions that may arise.

See complete prescribing literature for additional information.

CHART 69 : VITAMIN A SUPPLEMENTS (CAROTENES)

EXAMPLES:

AQUASOL-A BETA-CAROTENE VITAMIN A

INDICATIONS & EFFECTS:

Vitamin A deficiency and other conditions as determined by physician. Effects occur through vitamin replacement to aid in eye disorders, bone, skin, hair and teeth development.

DRUG-DISEASE PRECAUTIONS:

Hypervitaminosis, malabsorption, renal problems

DRUG-ALLERGY PRECAUTIONS:

Sensitivity to Vitamin A

PRECAUTIONS:

Have frequent check-ups especially if over 25,000 units of vitamin A daily. Excess may retard growth. Maintain balanced diet.

SIDE EFFECTS: Rare

REPORT: Nausea and vomiting, Night sweats, Dizziness, Cracking skin, Alopecia, Swelling of tongue, Jaundice, Bone pain, Loss of appetite

MONITOR: Mild nausea, Irritability, Headache, Edema, Skin irritation

*** PREGNANCY/NURSING/AGE/STORAGE/ABUSE PRECAUTIONS:**

Requirements of necessary vitamins are increased with pregnancy. Notify physician if pregnant or nursing. Excess may retard growth in young.

Interacting drugs may be used together in some conditions.

DRUG INTERACTIONS FOR: VITAMIN A SUPPLEMENTS (CAROTENES)

+ Cholestyramine, - **May seriously** decrease effects of former drug, take Vitamin A one hour before or two hours after.
+ Oral contraceptives - May increase effects of former drug
+ Anticoagulants - May decrease effects of latter drug with large doses of Vitamin A

FOOD/NUTRIENT INTERACTIONS:

+ Fish, liver, milk, cheese, carrots - May increase levels of carotenes and vitamin A and should be included in a balanced diet.
+ Mineral oil, fad diets - **May seriously** decrease effects of former drug

RX LABEL PRECAUTIONS:

Take only as directed with food. DO NOT double dose.

***Store all medicines out of childrens reach, away from heat and direct sunlight. Discard old/outdated medications.**
Inform physician(s)/pharmacist of all current medications and any questions that may arise.

See complete prescribing literature for additional information.

CHART 70 : VITAMIN B-1 SUPPLEMENTS (THIAMINE)

EXAMPLES:

BETALIN BETALIN-S THIAMINE VITAMIN B-1

INDICATIONS & EFFECTS:

Beriberi, Thiamine deficiency and other conditions as determined by physician. Effects occur through vitamin replacement to aid in growth, nervous system functions, muscles and heart.

DRUG-DISEASE PRECAUTIONS:

Wernicke's syndrome precautions

DRUG-ALLERGY PRECAUTIONS:

Sensitivity to Thiamine of B-1

PRECAUTIONS:

Unstable in alkaline solution, Carbonates, Citrates, Sulfites. Maintain balanced diet

SIDE EFFECTS: Rare

REPORT: Swelling, Difficult breathing, Tightness of throat
MONITOR: Feeling of warmth, Itching, Weakness, Nausea, Restlessness, Sweating

*** PREGNANCY/NURSING/AGE/STORAGE/ABUSE PRECAUTIONS:**

Inform physician if pregnant or nursing. Requirements of necessary vitamins are increased with pregnancy.

Interacting drugs may be used together in some conditions.

DRUG INTERACTIONS FOR: VITAMIN B-1 SUPPLEMENTS (THIAMINE)

+ Alcohol - **May seriously** effects of former drug

FOOD/NUTRIENT INTERACTIONS:

+ Cereals, milk, eggs, liver, pork, peaches, green vegetables, corn - May increase levels of Thiamine and should be included in a balanced diet.
+ Fad diets - May severely decrease levels of Thiamine

RX LABEL PRECAUTIONS:

Take with food.

***Store all medicines out of childrens reach, away from heat and direct sunlight. Discard old/outdated medications.**
Inform physician(s)/pharmacist of all current medications and any questions that may arise.

See complete prescribing literature for additional information.

CHART 71 : VITAMIN B-3 SUPPLEMENTS (NIACIN)

EXAMPLES: Also see Chart 29

NIACIN NICOBID NICOLAR NICOTINIC ACID VITAMIN B-3

INDICATIONS & EFFECTS:

Pellagra, Hyperlipidemia, and other conditions as determined by physician. Effects occur through vitamin replacement to aid in skin, nerves, digestive system, cholesterol control and vertigo.

DRUG-DISEASE PRECAUTIONS:

Various bleeding conditions, Hepatic Disease, Peptic ulcer, Diabetes

DRUG-ALLERGY PRECAUTIONS:

Sensitivity to any ingredients or Niacinamide

PRECAUTIONS:

May elevate blood sugar level or cause dizziness. Check with physician before discontinuing. Persistent flushing of skin may be decreased by one aspirin tablet 30 minutes before Niacin. Maintain balanced diet

SIDE EFFECTS: Rare

REPORT: Allergic reaction, Rash, Itching, Difficult breathing, Persistent diarrhea or irregular heartbeat, Frequent urination or thirst, Joint pain, Swelling, Fever

MONITOR: Dizziness, Faintness, Feeling of warmth, Flushing or tingling of skin, Headache, Nausea

*** PREGNANCY/NURSING/AGE/STORAGE/ABUSE PRECAUTIONS:**

Inform physician if pregnant or nursing, requirements of necessary vitamins are increased with pregnancy. Not recommended in children under two years old.

Interacting drugs may be used together in some conditions.

DRUG INTERACTIONS FOR: VITAMIN B-3 SUPPLEMENTS (NIACIN)

+ Chenodiol, Isoniazid - May decrease effectiveness of former drug
+ Lovastatin, Pravastatin, Simvastatin - **May seriously** increase side effects of latter drug

FOOD/NUTRIENT INTERACTIONS:

+ Eggs, meat, poultry, dairy products, tuna, peanut butter, enriched bread - May increase levels of Niacin and should be included in a balanced diet
+ Fad diets - May severely decrease levels of Niacin

RX LABEL PRECAUTIONS:

Take with food.

***Store all medicines out of childrens reach, away from heat and direct sunlight. Discard old/outdated medications.**
Inform physician(s)/pharmacist of all current medications and any questions that may arise.

See complete prescribing literature for additional information.

CHART 72 : VITAMIN B-6 SUPPLEMENTS (PYRIDOXINE)

EXAMPLES:

HEXA-BETALIN PYRIDOXINE VITABEE 6 VITAMIN B-6

INDICATIONS & EFFECTS:

Certain anemias, Deficiency states, TPN supplementation and other conditions as determined by physician. Effects occur through vitamin replacement to aid in proteins, amino acids, red blood cells and fat metabolism.

DRUG-DISEASE PRECAUTIONS:

Malabsorption syndromes

DRUG-ALLERGY PRECAUTIONS:

Sensitivity to any ingredients

PRECAUTIONS:

Megadoses may cause sensory problems. Avoid megadoses unless otherwise directed by a physician. Maintain balanced diet.

SIDE EFFECTS: Rare

REPORT: Numbness, Clumsiness

MONITOR: Nausea

*** PREGNANCY/NURSING/AGE/STORAGE/ABUSE PRECAUTIONS:**

Inform physician if pregnant or nursing, large doses not advised. Essential vitamin requirements are increased with pregnancy.

Interacting drugs may be used together in some conditions.

DRUG INTERACTIONS FOR: VITAMIN B-6 SUPPLEMENTS **(PYRIDOXINE)**

+ Levodopa (plain) - May decrease effectiveness of latter drug (combinations of Levodopa and carbidopa-sinemet) will not interact
+ Estrogens, Oral contraceptives, Isoniazid, Penicillamine, Steroids, Chloramphenicol, Cycloserine, Immunosuppressants, Peripheral vasodilators - May decrease effects of former drug (requirements may be increased)

FOOD/NUTRIENT INTERACTIONS:

+ Green leafy vegetables, beans, cereals, liver, beef, eggs, fish and potatoes - May increase levels of Pyridoxine and should be included in a balanced diet.

RX LABEL PRECAUTIONS:

Take with food, avoid megadoses.

***Store all medicines out of childrens reach, away from heat and direct sunlight. Discard old/outdated medications.**
Inform physician(s)/pharmacist of all current medications and any questions that may arise.

See complete prescribing literature for additional information.

CHART 73 : VITAMIN B-12 SUPPLEMENTS (CYANOCOBALAMIN)

EXAMPLES:

BETALIN 12 CYANOCOBALAMIN REDISOL RUBRAMIN-PC VITAMIN B-12

INDICATIONS & EFFECTS:

Pernicious anemia, Deficiency states, and other conditions as determined by physician. Effects occur through vitamin replacement to aid growth, nerves, blood cells and absorption disorders.

DRUG-DISEASE PRECAUTIONS:

Folic acid and B12 may mask pernicious anemia, Leber's disease, Malabsorption states

DRUG-ALLERGY PRECAUTIONS:

Sensitivity to any ingredients or cobalamins

PRECAUTIONS:

Folic acid and B12 may mask pernicious anemia. Potassium level may be severely decreased when first treated for megaloblastic anemia, injection may contain benzyl alcohol - avoid in newborn. Maintain balanced diet

SIDE EFFECTS: Rare

REPORT: Rash, Difficult breathing, Severe itching

MONITOR: Diarrhea, Minor skin irritation

*** PREGNANCY/NURSING/AGE/STORAGE/ABUSE PRECAUTIONS:**

Inform physician if pregnant or nursing. Requirements of necessay vitamins are increased with pregnancy. Avoid injectable form in newborn if containing benzyl alcohol.

Interacting drugs may be used together in some conditions.

DRUG INTERACTIONS FOR: VITAMIN B-12 SUPPLEMENTS **(CYANOCOBALAMIN)**

+ Alcohol, Colchicine, Cholestyramine, Neomycin - May decrease effects of former drug
+ Antibiotics - May decrease effects of former drug; take one hour apart
+ Folic Acid, Ascorbic Acid (large doses) - May decrease effects of former drug; take one hour apart

FOOD/NUTRIENT INTERACTIONS:

+ Fish, egg yolk, milk, fermented cheeses - May increase levels of B12 and should be included in a balanced diet.
+ Fad diets - May severely decrease levels of B12

RX LABEL PRECAUTIONS:

Take with food.

***Store all medicines out of childrens reach, away from heat and direct sunlight. Discard old/outdated medications.**
Inform physician(s)/pharmacist of all current medications and any questions that may arise.

See complete prescribing literature for additional information.

CHART 74 : VITAMIN C SUPPLEMENTS (ASCORBIC ACID)

EXAMPLES:

ASCORBIC ACID ASCORBICAP CE-VI-SOL CECON CEVALIN VITAMIN C

INDICATIONS & EFFECTS:

Deficiency states, Scurvy, and other conditions as determined by physician. Effects occur through vitamin replacement to aid in growth, blood cells, bone marrow and possible increased resistance.

DRUG-DISEASE PRECAUTIONS:

Sickle cell anemia, High doses of Vitamin C with Diabetes, G6PD, Kidney stones

DRUG-ALLERGY PRECAUTIONS:

Sensitivity to any ingredients

PRECAUTIONS:

Long use of 1000+mg. may lead to kidney stones, if not adequately hydrated, avoid megadoses unless directed by a physician, Urinary glucose tests may be affected, and occult blood tests. Maintain balanced diet.

SIDE EFFECTS: Rare

REPORT: Side or lower back pain, Diarrhea
MONITOR: Nausea, Cramps, Flushing of skin

*** PREGNANCY/NURSING/AGE/STORAGE/ABUSE PRECAUTIONS:**

Inform physician if pregnant or nursing. Essential vitamin requirements are increased in pregnancy, but megadoses are not recommended.

Interacting drugs may be used together in some conditions.

DRUG INTERACTIONS FOR: VITAMIN C SUPPLEMENTS **(ASCORBIC ACID)**

+ Deferoxamine - **May seriously** increase the side effects of latter drug
+ Mexiletine - May decrease effects of latter drug
+ Barbiturates, Primidone, Salicylates - May decrease effects of former drug (requirements may be increased)

FOOD/NUTRIENT INTERACTIONS:

+ Citrus fruits, green vegetables, tomatoes, potatoes - May increase levels of Vitamin C and should be included in a balanced diet.
+ Smoking, fad diets - **May seriously** decrease levels of Vitamin C

RX LABEL PRECAUTIONS:

Take with food.

***Store all medicines out of childrens reach, away from heat and direct sunlight. Discard old/outdated medications.**
Inform physician(s)/pharmacist of all current medications and any questions that may arise.

See complete prescribing literature for additional information.

CHART 75 : VITAMIN D & RELATED DRUGS

EXAMPLES:

CALCIFEROL CALCITRIOL DELTALIN DHT DIHYDROTACHYSTE ERGOCALCIFEROL HYTAKEROL ROCALTROL VITAMIN D

INDICATIONS & EFFECTS:

Hypocalcemia, Hypophosphatemia, Rickets, Tetany, Deficiency states, Extended lack of sunlight and other conditions as determined by physician. Effects occur through vitamin replacement to aid in growth, bones, calcium metabolism and teeth.

DRUG-DISEASE PRECAUTIONS:

Hypercalcemia, Hyperphosphatemia, Renal or Cardiac impairment, Arteriosclerosis

DRUG-ALLERGY PRECAUTIONS:

Sensitivity to any ingredients

PRECAUTIONS:

Avoid magnesium antacids with calciferol, calcitriol. Avoid megadoses. Have frequent check-ups, avoid non-prescription calcium unless otherwise directed. Maintain balanced diet.

SIDE EFFECTS: Rare

REPORT: Constipation, Diarrhea, Headache, Metal taste, Increased thirst or dry mouth, Unusual tiredness, Muscle or bone pain, Increased blood pressure, Irregular heartbeat, Vision problems

MONITOR: Itching, Nausea or vomiting, Mood changes

*** PREGNANCY/NURSING/AGE/STORAGE/ABUSE PRECAUTIONS:**

Best to avoid supplements in pregnancy unless otherwise directed, infants may be more susceptible to effects.

Interacting drugs may be used together in some conditions.

DRUG INTERACTIONS FOR: VITAMIN D & RELATED DRUGS
ALL PRODUCTS

+ Aluminum antacids, anticonvulsants, Barbiturates, Primidone, Cholestyramine, Colestipol, Sucralfate - May decrease effects of former drug
+ Calcitonin - May decrease effects of latter drug
+ Calcium, Diuretics Thiazide - May increase effects of former drug

CALCIFEROL & CALCITRIOL PRODUCTS - In addition

+ Magnesium antacids - **May seriously** increase effects of magnesium

FOOD/NUTRIENT INTERACTIONS:

+ Fish, fortified milk and bread - May increase Vitamin D levels and should be included in a balanced diet
+ Fad diets - May severely decrease Vitamin D levels
+ Calcium, Phosphorus - **May seriously** increase effects of former drug

RX LABEL PRECAUTIONS:

Take with food. Do Not double dose.

***Store all medicines out of childrens reach, away from heat and direct sunlight. Discard old/outdated medications.**
Inform physician(s)/pharmacist of all current medications and any questions that may arise.

See complete prescribing literature for additional information.

CHART 76 : VITAMIN E SUPPLEMENTS (ALPHA TOCOPHEROL)

EXAMPLES:

ALPHA TOCOPHEROL AQUASOL E EPROLIN VITAMIN E

INDICATIONS & EFFECTS:

Deficiency state, TPN nutrition, and other conditions as determined by physician. Effects occur through vitamin replacement to aid in growth, blood cells and protects against oxidation.

DRUG-DISEASE PRECAUTIONS:

Hypoprothrombinemia, Iron deficiency anemia

DRUG-ALLERGY PRECAUTIONS:

Sensitivity to any ingredients

PRECAUTIONS:

Avoid megadoses unless directed by physician. Maintain balanced diet.

SIDE EFFECTS: Rare

REPORT: Vision problems, Dizziness, Headache

MONITOR: Nausea, Tiredness or weakness

* **PREGNANCY/NURSING/AGE/STORAGE/ABUSE PRECAUTIONS:**

Inform physician if pregnant or nursing; premature infants may require supplements. Avoid injectables containing benzyl alcohol in newborns.

Interacting drugs may be used together in some conditions.

DRUG INTERACTIONS FOR: VITAMIN E SUPPLEMENTS **(ALPHA TOCOPHEROL)**

+ Iron - May decrease effects of latter drug
+ Antacids, Cholestyramine, Colestipol, Mineral oil, Sucralfate - May decrease effects of former drug - Take vitamin one hour before latter drug
+ Anticoagulants - May increase effects of latter drug

FOOD/NUTRIENT INTERACTIONS:

+ Vegetable oils, whole grain cereals, green leafy vegetables - May increase Vitamin E levels and should be included in a balanced diet.
+ Fad diets - May severely decrease levels of Vitamin E

RX LABEL PRECAUTIONS:

Take with food.

***Store all medicines out of childrens reach, away from heat and direct sunlight. Discard old/outdated medications.**
Inform physician(s)/pharmacist of all current medications and any questions that may arise.

See complete prescribing literature for additional information.

CHART 77 : VITAMIN FOLIC ACID & RELATED DRUGS

EXAMPLES:

BC FOLIC PLUS BEROCCA-PLUS FOLIC ACID FOLVITE NATABEC-FA NATABEC-RX NATALINS-RX PRAMET-FA PRAMILET-FA

INDICATIONS & EFFECTS:

Megaloblastic anemia, malabsorption, deficiency, and other conditions as determined by physician. Effects occur through vitamin replacement to aid in blood cells, nervous system, growth and anemia.

DRUG-DISEASE PRECAUTIONS:

Pernicious anemia

DRUG-ALLERGY PRECAUTIONS:

Sensitivity to any ingredients

PRECAUTIONS:

Maintain balanced diet and avoid megadoses unless otherwise directed by physician. Injectable form may contain benzyl alcohol, avoid in newborn.

SIDE EFFECTS: Rare

REPORT: Allergic reaction, Shortness of breath, Fever, Skin rash

MONITOR: Nausea

*** PREGNANCY/NURSING/AGE/STORAGE/ABUSE PRECAUTIONS:**

Inform physician if pregnant or nursing. Essential vitamin requirements are increased in pregnancy. Avoid injectable form in newborn if containing benzyl alcohol.

Interacting drugs may be used together in some conditions.

DRUG INTERACTIONS FOR: FOLIC ACID & RELATED DRUGS

+ Analgesics (long-term), Phenytoin (hydantoins), Estrogens, Antibiotics, Cholestyramine, Sulfonamides, Sulfasalazine, Methotrexate, Triamterene, Trimethoprim - May decrease effects of former drug

FOOD/NUTRIENT INTERACTIONS:

+ Green vegetables, cereal, potatoes, fruits, liver - May increase folic acid levels and should be included in a balanced diet.
+ Fad diets - **May seriously** decrease folic acid levels

RX LABEL PRECAUTIONS:

Take with food. Do not double dose.

***Store all medicines out of childrens reach, away from heat and direct sunlight. Discard old/outdated medications.**
Inform physician(s)/pharmacist of all current medications and any questions that may arise.

See complete prescribing literature for additional information.

CHART 78 : VITAMIN K SUPPLEMENTS

EXAMPLES:
MENADIOL MEPHYTON PHYTONADIONE SYNKAYVITE

INDICATIONS & EFFECTS:
Hypoprothrombinemia, Coagulation disorders, TPN supplementation and other conditions as determined by physician. Effects occur through vitamin replacement to aid in growth, development and decrease abnormal bleeding.

DRUG-DISEASE PRECAUTIONS:
G6PD deficiency, Hepatic disfunction

DRUG-ALLERGY PRECAUTIONS:
Sensitivity to any ingredients

PRECAUTIONS:
Have frequent check-ups and prothrombin tests, Maintain balanced diet

SIDE EFFECTS: Rare
REPORT: Allergic reaction, flushing
MONITOR: Unusual taste

*** PREGNANCY/NURSING/AGE/STORAGE/ABUSE PRECAUTIONS:**
Inform physician if pregnant or nursing; avoid in premature infant, caution in newborn and children.

Interacting drugs may be used together in some conditions.

DRUG INTERACTIONS FOR: VITAMIN K SUPPLEMENTS

+ Anticoagulants - **May seriously** decrease effects of latter drug
+ Antibiotics, Quinidine, Quinine, Salicylates, Sulfonamides, Cholestyramine, Colestipol, Sucralfate - May decrease effects of former drug

FOOD/NUTRIENT INTERACTIONS:

+ Leafy green vegetables, meats, dairy products - May increase Vitamin K levels and should be included in a balanced diet.
+ Fad Diets, Mineral Oil - May decrease Vitamin K levels

RX LABEL PRECAUTIONS:

Take with food. Do not double dose.

***Store all medicines out of childrens reach, away from heat and direct sunlight. Discard old/outdated medications.**
Inform physician(s)/pharmacist of all current medications and any questions that may arise.

See complete prescribing literature for additional information.

CHART 79 : VITAMINS & MINERALS

EXAMPLES: (See also specific Vitamin charts)

ADEFLOR BC FOLIC PLUS BEROCCA-PLUS CEFOL FERO-GRAD FERROUS SULFATE FEOSOL IBERET LURIDE NATABEC-RX NATALINS-RX POLY-VITES PRAMET-FA PRAMILET-FA THERAGRAN-M TRIHEMIC TRINSICON VITRON

INDICATIONS & EFFECTS:

Essential for enzymes and regulating physiological functions, Growth, Central nervous system, Tissue, Bones, and other conditions as determined by physician. Effects occur through vitamin and mineral replacement through a balanced diet, preferably, or supplementation.

DRUG-DISEASE PRECAUTIONS:

Certain cardiac, pulmonary or renal conditions

DRUG-ALLERGY PRECAUTIONS:

Sensitivity to any ingredients

PRECAUTIONS:

Avoid alcohol, Maintain balanced diet and avoid megadoses unless otherwise directed by physician. Injectable form may contain benzyl alcohol, avoid in newborn.

SIDE EFFECTS: Rare

REPORT: Allergic reaction, Shortness of breath, Fever, Skin rash
MONITOR: Nausea

*** PREGNANCY/NURSING/AGE/STORAGE/ABUSE PRECAUTIONS:**

Inform physician if pregnant or nursing. Essential vitamin and mineral requirements are increased in pregnancy. Avoid injectable forms containing benzyl alcohol in newborns.

Interacting drugs may be used together in some conditions.

DRUG INTERACTIONS FOR: MINERALS

ALL PRODUCTS

+ Alcohol - **May seriously** decrease effects of former mineral

CALCIUM

+ Iron, Tetracyclines - **May seriously** decrease effects of latter drug. Take as far apart as possible.

COPPER

+ Fiber, Megadoses of Vit C or Zinc - May decrease effects of former drug

FLUORIDE

+ Antacids (aluminum, calcium) - **May seriously** decrease effects of former drug

IODINE

+ Lithium - **May seriously** increase effects of former drug

IRON - FERROUS SULFATE

+ Fluroquinolones, Tetracyclines, Zinc - **May seriously** decrease effects of latter drug. Take as far apart as possible.
+ Levodopa, Methyldopa - May decrease effects of latter drug
+ Penicillamine - May increase side effects of latter drug
+ Antacids (carbonates), Caffeine, Cimetidine, Sulfasalazine - May decrease effects of former drug

MAGNESIUM

+ Ketoconazole, Tetracyclines - **May seriously** decrease effects of latter drug
+ Megadoses Vitamins A, E, K - May decrease effects of former mineral

ZINC

+ Fluroquinolones, Tetracyclines - **May seriously** decrease effects of latter drug. Take as far apart as possible.
+ Folic Acid, Iron - **May seriously** decrease effects of former mineral

FOOD/NUTRIENT INTERACTIONS:

+ Fad diets - **May seriously** decrease mineral & vitamin levels

RX LABEL PRECAUTIONS:

Take with food as directed. Maintain a balanced diet.

***Store all medicines out of childrens reach, away from heat and direct sunlight. Discard old/outdated medications. Inform physician or pharmacist of all current medications and any questions. See complete prescribing literature for additional information.**

INDEX

A

INDEX

ANHYDRON CH.37 CYCLOTHIAZIDE
ANISOTROPINE CH.12 VALPIN-50
ANSAID CH.53 FLURBIPROFEN
ANTACIDS CH.10
ANTIANXIETY + SEDATIVE AGENTS CH.11
ANTICHOLINERGIC & ANTISPASMODICS CH.12
ANTICOAGULANTS CH.13
ANTICONVULSANTS 1 CH.14
ANTICONVULSANTS 2 CH.15
ANTIDEPRESSANTS CH.16
ANTIHISTAMINE & DECONGESTANTS CH.18
ANTIHISTAMINES CH.17
ANTIMETABOLITE AGENTS CH.5
ANTIPARKINSONS CH.19
ANTIULCER + H2 BLOCKERS CH.20
ANTURANE CH.43 SULFINPYRAZONE
APAP CH.3 ACETAMINOPHEN
APAP/CODEINE CH.51 + see ACETAMINOPHEN, CODEINE
APRESAZIDE CH.56 + see HYDRALAZINE, HYDROCHLOROTHIAZIDE
APRESOLINE CH.56 HYDRALAZINE
APRESOLINE-ESIDIX CH.56 + see HYDRALAZINE, HYDROCHLOROTHIAZIDE
APROBARBITAL CH.23 ALURATE
AQUASOL-E CH.76 ALPHA TOCOPHEROL
AQUASOL-A CH.69 VITAMIN A
AQUATENSEN CH.37 METHYCLOTHIAZIDE
ARISTO-PAK CH.60 TRIAMCINOLONE
ARISTOCORT CH.60 TRIAMCINOLONE
ARLIDIN CH.67 NYLIDRIN
ARMOUR THYROID CH.64 THYROID
ARRHYTHMIC AGENTS 1 CH.21
ARRHYTHMIC AGENTS 2 CH.22
ARTHROPAN CH.58 CHOLINE SALICYLATE
ASA CH.58 ASPIRIN
ASA/CODEINE CH.51 + see ASPIRIN, CODEINE
ASA/OXYCODONE CH.51 PERCODAN
ASBRON-G CH.63 + see THEOPHYLLINE, GUAIFENESIN
ASCORBIC ACID CH.74 VITAMIN C
ASCORBICAP CH.74 VITAMIN C
ASCRIPTIN CH.58 BUFFERED ASPIRIN
ASENDIN CH.16 AMOXAPINE

INDEX

C

INDEX

CEFAMANDOLE CH.28 MANDOL
CEFANEX CH.28 CEPHALEXIN
CEFIXIME CH.28 SUPRAX
CEFIZOX CH.28 CEFTIZOXIME
CEFOL CH.79 VITAMINS & MINERALS
CEFOL CH.79 MULTIVITAMIN
CEFONICID CH.28 MONOCID
CEFOTAXIME CH.28 CLAFORAN
CEFOXITIN CH.28 MEFOXIN
CEFPROZIL CH.28 CEFZIL
CEFTAZIDIME CH.28 CEPTAZ
CEFTAZIDIME CH.28 FORTAZ
CEFTAZIDIME CH.28 TAZICEF
CEFTIN CH.28 CEFUROXIME
CEFTIZOXIME CH.28 CEFIZOX
CEFTRIAXONE CH.28 ROCEPHIN
CEFUROXIME CH.28 CEFTIN
CEFUROXIME CH.28 ZINACEF
CEFZIL CH.28 CEFPROZIL
CELESTONE CH.60 BETAMETHASONE
CELONTIN CH.15 METHSUXIMIDE
CENTRAX CH.11 PRAZEPAM
CEPHALEXIN CH.28 CEFANEX
CEPHALEXIN CH.28 KEFLET
CEPHALEXIN CH.28 KEFLEX
CEPHALEXIN HCL CH.28 KEFTAB
CEPHALOSPORINS CH.28
CEPHRADINE CH.28 VELOSEF
CEPTAZ CH.28 CEFTAZIDIME
CERESPAN CH.67 PAPAVERINE
CERUBIDINE CH.52 DAUNORUBICIN
CEVALIN CH.74 VITAMIN C
CHERACOL CH.32 + see GUAIFENESIN, CODEINE
CHLORAL HYDRATE CH.59 CHLORAL HYDRATE
CHLORAL HYDRATE CH.59 CHLORAL HYDRATE
CHLORAL HYDRATE CH.59 NOCTEC
CHLORAMBUCIL CH.5 LEUKERAN
CHLORDIAZEPOXIDE, CLINDINIUM CH.12 CLINDEX
CHLORDIAZEPOXIDE, CLIDINIUM CH.12 LIBRAX
CHLORDIAZEPOXIDE, AMITRIPTYLINE CH.16 LIMBITROL
CHLORDIAZEPOXIDE CH.11 LIBRITABS
CHLORDIAZEPOXIDE CH.11 LIBRIUM

CHLORPHENIRAMINE, PHENYLEPHRINE, DM, GG CH.32
DONATUSSIN
CHLORPHENIRAMINE, PSEUDOEPHEDRINE, CODEINE CH.32
NOVAHISTINE DH
CHLORPHENIRAMINE, CODEINE CH.32 PENNTUSS
CHLORPHENIRAMINE, PSEUDOEPHEDRINE, CODEINE CH.32
RYNA-C
CHLORPHENIRAMINE, PHENYLPROPANOLAMINE, DM CH.32
TRIAMINICOL
CHLORPHENIRAMINE, PHENYLEPHRINE, PPA, DM CH.32
TUSQUELIN
CHLORPHENIRAMINE, CODEINE, GUAIFENESIN CH.32 TUSSAR-2
CHLORPHENIRAMINE, PSEUDOEPHEDRINE, DM CH.32
TUSSAR-DM
CHLORPHENIRAMINE, CODEINE, GUAIFENESIN CH.32 TUSSAR-SF
CHLORPROMAZINE CH.65 THORAZINE
CHLORPROPAMIDE CH.34 DIABINESE
CHLORPROTHIXENE CH.65 TARACTAN
CHLORTHALIDONE CH.37 HYGROTON
CHLORTHALIDONE CH.37 THALITONE
CHLORTRIMETON CH.17 CHLORPHENIRAMINE
CHLORZOXAZONE CH.50 PARAFLEX
CHLORZOXAZONE CH.50 PARAFON FORTE D
CHOCOLATE CH.1 CAFFEINE PRODUCT
CHOLEDYL CH.63 OXTRIPHYLLINE
CHOLESTEROL AGENTS CH.29
CHOLESTYRAMINE CH.29 QUESTRAN
CHOLINE MAGNESIUM SALICYLATES CH.58 TRILISATE
CHOLINE SALICYLATE CH.58 ARTHROPAN
CIBALITH-S CH.45 LITHIUM
CIGARETTES CH.1 NICOTINE
CIGARS CH.1 NICOTINE
CIMETIDINE CH.20 TAGAMET
CIN QUIN CH.21 QUINIDINE
CINOBAC CH.41 CINOXACIN
CINOXACIN CH.41 CINOBAC
CIPRO CH.41 CIPROFLOXACIN
CIPROFLOXACIN CH.41 CIPRO
CISPLATIN CH.5 PLATINOL
CLAFORAN CH.28 CEFOTAXIME
CLARITHROMYCIN CH.39 BIAXIN
CLEMASTINE CH.17 TAVIST

COMPAL CH.51 + see DIHYDROCODONE, ACETAMINOPHEN
COMPAZINE CH.65 PROCHLORPERAZINE
CONAR CH.32 + see PHENYLEPHRINE, DEXTROMETHORPHAN
CONAR EXP CH.32 + see PHENYLEPHRINE, DM, GUIAFENESIN
CONAR-A CH.32 + see PHENYLEPHRINE, DM,
GUAIFENESIN, APAP
CONJ ESTROGEN CH.40 ESTROGENS CONJUGATED
CONSTANT-T CH.63 THEOPHYLLINE
CONTAC CH.18 CHLORPHENIRAMINE, PHENYLPROPANOLAMINE
COPPER CH.79 MINERAL
CORDARONE CH.22 AMIODARONE
CORGARD CH.24 NADALOL
CORTEF CH.60 HYDROCORTISONE
CORTISONE CH.60 CORTONE
CORTONE CH.60 CORTISONE
CORZIDE CH.24 + see NADALOL, HYDROCHLOROTHIAZIDE
COSMEGEN CH.52 DACTINOMYCIN
COUGH & COLD EXPECTORANTS CH.31
COUGH & COLD SUPPRESSANTS CH.32
COUMADIN CH.13 WARFARIN SODIUM
CPM W/PPA CH.18 CHLORPHENIRAMINE, PHENYLPROPANOLAMINE
CPM, EPHEDRINE, PHENYLEPHRINE, CARBETAPENTANE CH.32
RYNATUSS
CPM, PHENYLEPHRINE, CODEINE, POTASSIUM IODIDE CH.31
PEDIACOF
CPM, PHENYLPROPANOLAMINE, PHENYLEPHRINE, P-TOLOX.
CH.18 NALDECON
CRYSTODIGIN CH.35 DIGITOXIN
CYANOCOBALAMIN CH.73 VITAMIN B-12
CYCLANDELATE CH.67 CYCLOSPASMOL
CYCLOBENZAPRINE CH.50 FLEXERIL
CYCLOPHOSPHAMIDE CH.5 CYTOXAN
CYCLOPHOSPHAMIDE CH.5 NEOSAR
CYCLOSPASMOL CH.67 CYCLANDELATE
CYCLOTHIAZIDE CH.37 ANHYDRON
CYCRIN CH.40 MEDROXYPROGESTERONE
CYLERT CH.30 PEMOLINE
CYPROHEPTADINE CH.17 PERIACTIN
CYSTOSPAZ CH.12 + see HYOSCYAMINE, BUTABARBITAL
CYTARABINE CH.5 CYTOSAR-U
CYTOMEL CH.64 LIOTHYRONINE
CYTOSAR-U CH.5 CYTARABINE

DEPAKOTE CH.14 DIVALPROEX
DEPO-ESTRADIOL CH.40 ESTRADIOL CYPIONATE
DEPO-MEDROL CH.60 METHYLPREDNISOLONE
DEPO-PROVERA CH.40 MEDROXYPROGESTERONE
DEPO-TESTADIOL CH.40 + see ESTRADIOL, TESTOSTERONE
DEPONIT CH.67 NITROGLYCERIN
DES CH.40 DIETHYLSTILBESTROL
DESERPIDINE CH.4 HARMONYL
DESERPIDINE, METHYCLOTHIAZIDE CH.4 ENDURONYL
DESIPRAMINE CH.16 NORPRAMIN
DESIPRAMINE CH.16 PERTOFRANE
DESOXYN CH.30 METHAMPHETAMINE
DESYREL CH.16 TRAZODONE
DEXAMETHASONE CH.60 DECADRON
DEXAMETHASONE CH.60 HEXADROL
DEXATRIM CH.33 PHENYLPROPANOLAMINE
DEXBROMPHENIRAMINE, PSEUDOEPHEDRINE CH.18 DISOBROM
DEXBROMPHENIRAMINE, PSEUDOEPHEDRINE CH.18 DISOPHROL
DEXBROMPHENIRAMINE, PSEUDOEPHEDRINE CH.18 DRIXORAL
DEXCHLORPHENIRAMINE CH.17 POLARAMINE
DEXCHLORPHENIRAMINE CH.17 POLARGEN TD
DEXEDRINE CH.30 DEXTROAMPHETAMINE
DEXTROAMPHETAMINE CH.30 DEXEDRINE
DEXTROMETHORPHAN CH.32 BENYLIN DM
DEXTROMETHORPHAN CH.32 DELSYM
DHT CH.75 DIHYDROTACHYSTEROL
DI-GEL CH.10 ALUMINUM, MAGNESIUM, SIMETHICONE
DIABETA CH.34 GLYBURIDE
DIABETIC AGENTS CH.34
DIABINESE CH.34 CHLORPROPAMIDE
DIAMOX CH.27 ACETAZOLAMIDE
DIAZEPAM CH.11 VALIUM
DIAZEPAM CH.11 VALRELEASE
DICHLORPHENAMIDE CH.27 DARANIDE
DICLOFENAC CH.53 VOLTAREN
DICLOXACILLIN CH.55 DYCILL
DICLOXACILLIN CH.55 DYNAPEN
DICOUMAROL CH.13 DICUMAROL
DICUMAROL CH.13 DICOUMAROL
DICYCLOMINE CH.12 BENTYL
DIDEOXYCYTIDINE CH.68 DDC

DISOPHROL CH.18 DEXBROMPHENIRAMINE, PSEUDOEPHEDRINE
DISOPYRAMIDE CH.21 NORPACE
DISOPYRAMIDE CH.21 NORPACE CR
DIUCARDIN CH.37 HYDROFLUMETHIAZIDE
DIULO CH.37 METOLAZONE
DIUPRES CH.4 + see RESERPINE, CHLOROTHIAZIDE
DIURETICS POTASSIUM SPARING CH.36
DIURETICS THIAZIDE & LOOP CH.37
DIURIGEN W/R CH.4 + see RESERPINE, CHLOROTHIAZIDE
DIURIL CH.37 CHLOROTHIAZIDE
DIUTENSEN-R CH.4 + see RESERPINE, METHYLCLOTHIAZIDE
DIVALPROEX CH.14 DEPAKOTE
DM CH.32 DEXTROMETHORPHAN
DOLOBID CH.53 DIFLUNISAL
DOLOPHINE CH.51 METHADONE
DONATUSSIN CH.32 + see CHLORPHENIRAMINE, PHENYLEPHRINE, DM, GG
DONNATAL CH.12 + see ATROPINE, HYOSCYAMINE, SCOPOLAMINE, PB
DOPAR CH.19 LEVODOPA
DORIDEN CH.59 GLUTETHIMIDE
DORYX CH.62 DOXYCYCLINE
DOXAZOCIN CH.6 CARDURA
DOXEPIN CH.16 SINEQUAN
DOXORUBICIN CH.52 ADRIAMYCIN
DOXORUBICIN CH.52 RUBEX
DOXYCYCLINE CH.62 DORYX
DOXYCYCLINE CH.62 MONODOX
DOXYCYCLINE CH.62 VIBRAMYCIN
DOXYCYCLINE CH.62 VIBRATAB
DOXYLAMINE CH.17 UNISOM
DRAMAMINE CH.17 DIMENHYDRINATE
DRISTAN CH.18 CHLORPHENIRAMINE, PHENYLEPHRINE, ACETAMINOPHEN
DRIXORAL CH.18 DEXBROMPHENIRAMINE, PSEUDOEPHEDRINE
DTIC CH.52 DACARBAZINE
DUO-MEDIHALER CH.25 + see ISOPROTERENOL, PHENYLEPHRINE
DURAQUIN CH.21 QUINIDINE
DURICEF CH.28 CEFADROXIL
DYAZIDE CH.36 + see TRIAMTERENE, HYDROCHLOROTHIAZIDE
DYCILL CH.55 DICLOXACILLIN

ERGOCALCIFEROL CH.75 VITAMIN D
ERGOLOID MESYLATES CH.38 HYDERGINE
ERGOMAR CH.38 ERGOTAMINE
ERGONOVINE CH.38 ERGOTRATE
ERGOSTAT CH.38 ERGOTAMINE
ERGOTAMINE CH.38 ERGOMAR
ERGOTAMINE CH.38 ERGOSTAT
ERGOTAMINE CH.38 MEDIHALER-ERG
ERGOTAMINE & RELATED DRUGS CH.38
ERGOTAMINE, BELLADONNA, PB CH.38 BELLERGAL-S
ERGOTAMINE, CAFFEINE CH.38 CAFERGOT
ERGOTAMINE, CAFFEINE CH.38 ERGO-CAFF
ERGOTAMINE, CAFFEINE CH.38 WIGRAINE
ERGOTRATE CH.38 ERGONOVINE
ERY-TAB CH.39 ERYTHROMYCIN
ERY-TAB CH.39 ERYTHROMYCIN
ERYC CH.39 ERYTHROMYCIN
ERYPED CH.39 ERYTHROMYCIN ETHYLSUCCINATE
ERYTHRITYL TETRANITRATE CH.67 CARDILATE
ERYTHROCIN CH.39 ERYTHROMYCIN STEARATE
ERYTHROMYCIN CH.39 E-MYCIN
ERYTHROMYCIN CH.39 ERY-TAB
ERYTHROMYCIN CH.39 ERYC
ERYTHROMYCIN CH.39 PCE
ERYTHROMYCIN CH.39 ROBIMYCIN
ERYTHROMYCIN ESTOLATE CH.39 ILOSONE
ERYTHROMYCIN ETHYLSUCCINATE CH.39 E.E.S.
ERYTHROMYCIN ETHYLSUCCINATE CH.39 ERYPED
ERYTHROMYCIN STEARATE CH.39 ERYTHROCIN
ERYTHROMYCIN STEARATE CH.39 WYAMYCIN-S
ERYTHROMYCIN, SULFISOXAZOLE CH.61 EES/SULF
ERYTHROMYCIN, SULFISOXAZOLE CH.61 PEDIAZOLE
ERYTHROMYCINS CH.39
ESGIC CH.23 + see BUTALBITAL, ACETAMINOPHEN, CAFFEINE
ESIDRIX CH.37 HYDROCHLOROTHIAZIDE
ESIMIL CH.4 + see GUANETHIDINE, HYDROCHLOROTHIAZIDE
ESKALITH CH.45 LITHIUM CARBONATE
ESTAZOLAM CH.11 PROSOM
ESTINYL CH.40 ETHINYL ESTRADIOL
ESTRACE CH.40 ESTRADIOL
ESTRADERM CH.40 ESTRADIOL
ESTRADIOL CH.40 ESTRACE

FERANCEE CH.79 FERROUS SULFATE
FERMALOX CH.79 FERROUS SULFATE
FERO-FOL-500 CH.79 + see FERROUS SULFATE, VITAMINS
FERO-GRAD CH.79 VITAMINS & MINERALS
FERO-GRADUMT CH.79 FERROUS SULFATE
FERROUS FUMERATE CH.79 FEOSTAT
FERROUS SULFATE CH.79 MINERAL
FERROUS SULFATE CH.79 FER-IN-SOL
FERROUS SULFATE CH.79 FERMALOX
FERROUS SULFATE CH.79 FERO-GRADUMT
FERROUS SULFATE CH.79 MOL-IRON
FILIBON CH.79 MULTIVITAMIN
FIORGEN CH.23 + see BUTALBITAL, ACETAMINOPHEN, CAFFEINE
FIORICET CH.23 + see BUTALBITAL, ACETAMINOPHEN, CAFFEINE
FIORINAL CH.23 + see BUTALBITAL, ASPIRIN, CAFFEINE
FIORINAL+COD CH.23 + see BUTALBITAL, ASPIRIN, CAFFEINE, CODEINE
FLAGYL CH.49 METRONIDAZOLE
FLECAINIDE CH.22 TAMBOCOR
FLEXERIL CH.50 CYCLOBENZAPRINE
FLORINEF CH.60 FLUDROCORTISONE
FLOXIN CH.41 OFLOXACIN
FLOXURIDINE CH.5 FUDR
FLUCONAZOLE CH.42 DIFLUCAN
FLUCYTOSINE CH.42 ANCOBON
FLUDARA CH.5 FLUDARABINE
FLUDARABINE CH.5 FLUDARA
FLUDROCORTISONE CH.60 FLORINEF
FLUNISOLIDE CH.60 AEROBID
FLUNISOLIDE CH.60 NASALIDE
FLUORIDE CH.79 LURIDE
FLUORURACIL CH.5 ADRUCIL
FLUOXETINE CH.16 PROZAC
FLUOXYMESTERONE CH.9 HALOTESTIN
FLUPHENAZINE CH.65 PERMITIL
FLUPHENAZINE CH.65 PROLIXIN
FLURAZEPAM CH.11 DALMANE
FLURBIPROFEN CH.53 ANSAID
FLUROQUINOLONES & RELATED DRUGS CH.41
FLUTAMIDE CH.52 EULEXIN
FOLEX CH.47 METHOTREXATE
FOLIC ACID CH.77 FOLVITE

HYDRODIURIL CH.37 HYDROCHLOROTHIAZIDE
HYDROFLUMETHIAZIDE CH.37 DIUCARDIN
HYDROFLUMETHIAZIDE CH.37 SALURON
HYDROMORPHONE CH.51 DILAUDID
HYDROMOX CH.37 QUINETHAZONE
HYDROMOX-R CH.4 + see RESERPINE, QUINETHAZONE
HYDROPRES CH.4 + see RESERPINE, HYDROCHLOROTHIAZIDE
HYDROSERPINE CH.4 + see RESERPINE, HYDROCHLOROTHIAZIDE
HYDROXYUREA CH.52 HYDREA
HYDROXYZINE CH.17 ATARAX
HYDROXYZINE CH.17 VISTARIL
HYGROTON CH.37 CHLORTHALIDONE
HYLOREL CH.4 GUANADREL
HYOSCAMINE, SCOPOLAMINE, PHENOBARBITAL CH.12 BELLADENAL
HYOSCYAMINE CH.12 ANASPAZ
HYOSCYAMINE, BUTABARBITAL CH.12 CYSTOSPAZ
HYOSCYAMINE, CH.12 LEVSIN
HYOSCYAMINE, PHENOBARBITAL CH.12 LEVSINEX-PB
HYTAKEROL CH.75 DIHYDROTACHYSTEROL
HYTRIN CH.6 TERAZOCIN

I

IBERET CH.79 VITAMINS & MINERALS
IBERET-FOLIC CH.79 + see FERROUS SULFATE, VITAMINS
IBEROL-F CH.79 + see FERROUS SULFATE, VITAMINS
IBUPROFEN CH.53 ADVIL
IBUPROFEN CH.53 HALTRAN
IBUPROFEN CH.53 MOTRIN
IBUPROFEN CH.53 NUPRIN
IBUPROFEN CH.53 PEDIAPROFEN
IBUPROFEN CH.53 RUFEN
IDAMYCIN CH.52 IDARUBICIN
IDARUBICIN CH.52 IDAMYCIN
IFEX CH.5 IFOSFAMIDE
IFOSFAMIDE CH.5 IFEX
ILOSONE CH.39 ERYTHROMYCIN ESTOLATE
IMIPRAMINE CH.16 JANIMINE
IMIPRAMINE CH.16 TOFRANIL
INCREMIN CH.79 + see FERROUS SULFATE, VITAMINS
INDAPAMIDE CH.37 LOZOL
INDERAL CH.24 PROPRANOLOL
INDERAL LA CH.24 PROPRANOLOL

J

JANIMINE CH.16 IMIPRAMINE

K

K-DUR CH.57 POTASSIUM CHLORIDE
K-LOR POWDER CH.57 POTASSIUM CHLORIDE
K-LYTE-DS CH.57 POTASSIUM BICARBONATE
K-LYTE/CL CH.57 + see POTASSIUM BICARBONATE, POTASSIUM CHLORIDE
K-NORM CH.57 POTASSIUM CHLORIDE
K-PHOS CH.57 POTASSIUM PHOSPHATES
K-TABS CH.57 POTASSIUM CHLORIDE
KANAMYCIN CH.8 KANTREX
KANTREX CH.8 KANAMYCIN
KAOCHLOR CH.57 POTASSIUM CHLORIDE
KAON CH.57 POTASSIUM GLUCONATE
KAON-CL CH.57 POTASSIUM CHLORIDE
KAY CIEL CH.57 POTASSIUM CHLORIDE
KEFLET CH.28 CEPHALEXIN
KEFLEX CH.28 CEPHALEXIN
KEFTAB CH.28 CEPHALEXIN HCL
KENACORT CH.60 TRIAMCINOLONE
KENALOG CH.60 TRIAMCINOLONE
KETOCONAZOLE CH.42 NIZORAL
KETOPROFEN CH.53 ORUDIS
KETOROLAC CH.53 TORADOL
KIE CH.31 + see EPHEDRINE, POTASSIUM IODIDE
KINESED CH.12 + see ATROPINE, HYOSCYAMINE, SCOPOLAMINE, PB
KLONOPIN CH.11 CLONAZEPAM
KLOR-CON CH.57 POTASSIUM CHLORIDE
KLORVESS CH.57 + see POTASSIUM BICARBONATE, POTASSIUM CHLORIDE
KLOTRIX CH.57 POTASSIUM CHLORIDE
KOLYUM CH.57 + see POTASSIUM CHLORIDE, POTASSIUM GLUCOMATE

L

L-THYROXINE CH.64 LEVOTHYROXINE
LABETALOL CH.24 NORMODYNE
LABETALOL CH.24 TRANDATE
LABETALOL, HYDROCHLOROTHIAZIDE CH.24 NORMOZIDE
LABETALOL, HYDROCHLOROTHIAZIDE CH.24 TRANDATE HCT
LABID CH.63 THEOPHYLLINE
LANOXICAPS CH.35 DIGOXIN
LANOXIN CH.35 DIGOXIN

LITHIUM CARBONATE CH.45 LITHANE
LITHIUM CARBONATE CH.45 LITHOBID
LITHIUM CARBONATE CH.45 LITHONATE
LITHIUMS CH.45
LITHOBID CH.45 LITHIUM CARBONATE
LITHONATE CH.45 LITHIUM CARBONATE
LO/OVRAL CH.54 NORGESTREL, ETHINYL ESTRADIOL
LODINE CH.53 ETODOLAC
LOESTRIN CH.54 NORETHINDRONE, ETHINYL ESTRADIOL
LOGEN CH.51 DIPHENOXYLATE, ATROPINE
LOMEFLOXACIN CH.41 MAXAQUIN
LOMOTIL CH.51 DIPHENOXYLATE, ATROPINE
LOMUSTINE CH.5 CEENU
LONITEN CH.56 MINOXIDIL
LOPID CH.29 GEMFIBROZIL
LOPRESSOR CH.24 METOPROLOL
LOPRESSOR HCT CH.24 + see METOPROLOL, HYDROCHLOROTHIAZIDE
LOPURIN CH.43 ALLOPURINOL
LORAZEPAM CH.11 ATIVAN
LORCET CH.51 + see HYDROCODONE, ACETAMINOPHEN
LORELCO CH.29 PROBUCOL
LORTAB CH.51 + see HYDROCODONE, ACETAMINOPHEN
LORTAB ASA CH.51 + see HYDROCODONE, ASPIRIN
LOTENSIN CH.2 BENAZEPRIL
LOVASTATIN CH.29 MEVACOR
LOXAPINE CH.65 LOXITANE
LOXITANE CH.65 LOXAPINE
LOZOL CH.37 INDAPAMIDE
LUDIOMIL CH.16 MAPROTILINE
LUFYLLIN CH.63 DYPHYLLINE
LUFYLLIN-GG CH.63 + see DYPHYLLINE, GUAIFENESIN
LUMINAL CH.23 PHENOBARBITAL
LUPRON CH.52 LEUPROLIDE
LURIDE CH.79 FLUORIDE
LYSODREN CH.52 MITOTANE

M

MAALOX CH.10 ALUMINUM, MAGNESIUM
MAALOX PLUS CH.10 ALUMINUM, MAGNESIUM, SIMETHICONE
MACROBID CH.66 NITROFURANTOIN
MACRODANTIN CH.66 NITROFURANTOIN

MEPENZOLATE CH.12 CANTIL
MEPERIDINE CH.51 DEMEROL
MEPERIDINE, ACETAMINOPHEN CH.51 DEMEROL APAP
MEPHENYTOIN CH.14 MESANTOIN
MEPHOBARBITAL CH.23 MEBARAL
MEPHYTON CH.78 PHYTONADIONE
MEPROBAMATE CH.59 EQUANIL
MEPROBAMATE CH.59 MEPROSPAN
MEPROBAMATE CH.59 MILTOWN
MEPROBAMATE, ASA, ETHOHEPTAZINE, CH.59 EQUAGESIC
MEPROBAMATE, ASPIRIN CH.59 MICRAININ
MEPROSPAN CH.59 MEPROBAMATE
MERCAPTOPURINE CH.5 PURINETHOL
MESANTOIN CH.14 MEPHENYTOIN
MESORIDAZINE CH.65 SERENTIL
METAHYDRIN CH.37 TRICHLORMETHIAZIDE
METANDREN CH.9 METHYLTESTOSTERONE
METAPREL CH.25 METAPROTERENOL
METAPROTERENOL CH.25 ALUPENT
METAPROTERENOL CH.25 METAPREL
METATENSIN CH.4 + see RESERPINE, TRICHLORMETHIAZIDE
METAXALONE CH.50 SKELAXIN
METHACYCLINE CH.62 RONDOMYCIN
METHADONE CH.51 DOLOPHINE
METHAMPHETAMINE CH.30 DESOXYN
METHAZOLAMIDE CH.27 NEPTAZANE
METHDILAZINE CH.17 TACARYL
METHENAMINE HIPPURATE CH.66 HIPREX
METHENAMINE HIPPURATE CH.66 UREX
MANDELATE CH. 66 MANDELAMINE
METHERGINE CH. 38 METHYLERGONOVINE
METHOCARBAMOL CH.50 ROBAXIN
METHOCARBAMOL, ASPIRIN CH.50 ROBAXISAL
METHOTREXATE CH.47 MTX
METHOTREXATE CH.47 AMETHOPTERIN
METHOTREXATE CH.47 FOLEX
METHOTREXATE CH.47 MEXATE
METHOTREXATE CH.47 RHEUMATREX
METHSCOPOLAMINE CH.12 PAMINE
METHSUXIMIDE CH.15 CELONTIN
METHYCLOTHIAZIDE CH.37 AQUATENSEN
METHYCLOTHIAZIDE CH.37 ENDURON

MINOCIN CH.62 MINOCYCLINE
MINOCYCLINE CH.62 MINOCIN
MINOXIDIL CH.56 LONITEN
MISOPROSTOL CH.20 CYTOTEC
MITOMYCIN CH.52 MUTAMYCIN
MITOTANE CH.52 LYSODREN
MITOXANTRONE CH.52 NOVATRONE
MITRACIN CH.52 PLICAMYCIN
MIXTARD CH.34 INSULIN
MOBAN CH.65 MOLINDONE
MOBIDIN CH.58 MAGNESIUM SALICYLATE
MODICON CH.54 NORETHINDRONE, ETHINYL ESTRADIOL
MODURETIC CH.36 + see AMILORIDE, HYDROCHLOROTHIAZIDE
MOL-IRON CH.79 FERROUS SULFATE
MOLINDONE CH.65 MOBAN
MONO-GESIC CH.58 SALSALATE
MONOCID CH.28 CEFONICID
MONODOX CH.62 DOXYCYCLINE
MONOPRIL CH.2 FOSINOPRIL
MORICIZINE CH.22 ETHMOZINE
MORPHINE CH.51 MS CONTIN
MORPHINE CH.51 MSIR
MORPHINE CH.51 ORAMORPH
MORPHINE CH.51 ROXANOL
MOTOFEN CH.51 DIFENOXIN, ATROPINE
MOTRIN CH.53 IBUPROFEN
MOXALACTAM CH.28 MOXAM
MOXAM CH.28 MOXALACTAM
MS CONTIN CH.51 MORPHINE
MSIR CH.51 MORPHINE
MTX CH.47 METHOTREXATE
MULTICEBRIN CH.79 MULTIVITAMIN
MULTIVITAMIN CH.79 BEROCCA
MULTIVITAMIN CH.79 CEFOL
MULTIVITAMIN CH.79 THERAGRAN M
MULTIVITAMINS CH.79
MULVIDREN-F CH.79 + see VITAMINS, FLUORIDE
MUSCLE RELAXANTS SKELETAL CH.50
MUSTARGEN CH.5 MECHLORETHAMINE
MUTAMYCIN CH.52 MITOMYCIN
MYCOSTATIN CH.42 NYSTATIN
MYLANTA CH.10 ALUMINUM, MAGNESIUM, SIMETHICONE

NORINYL CH.54 NORETHINDRONE, MESTRANOL
NORISODRINE CH.25 ISOPROTERENOL
NORLESTRIN CH.54 NORETHINDRONE ACETATE, ETHINYL ESTRADIOL
NORLUTATE CH.40 NORETHINDRONE ACETATE
NORLUTIN CH.40 NORETHINDRONE
NORMODYNE CH.24 LABETALOL
NORMOZIDE CH.24 + see LABETALOL, HYDROCHLOROTHIAZIDE
NOROXIN CH.41 NORFLOXACIN
NORPACE CH.21 DISOPYRAMIDE
NORPACE CR CH.21 DISOPYRAMIDE
NORPRAMIN CH.16 DESIPRAMINE
NORTRIPTYLINE CH.16 AVENTYL
NORTRIPTYLINE CH.16 PAMELOR
NOVAFED CH.33 PSEUDOEPHEDRINE
NOVAFED A CH.18 CHLORPHENIRAMINE, PSEUDOEPHEDRINE
NOVAHISTINE CH.18 CHLORPHENIRAMINE, PHENYLEPHRINE
NOVAHISTINE DH CH.32 + see CHLORPHENIRAMINE, PSEUDOEPHEDRINE, CODEINE
NOVAHISTINE EXP CH.32 + see PSEUDOEPHEDRINE, CODEINE, GUIAFENESIN
NOVATRONE CH.52 MITOXANTRONE
NOVOLIN CH.34 INSULIN
NOVOLIN L,N,R CH.34 INSULIN
NUCOFED CH.32 + see PSEUDOEPHEDRINE, CODEINE
NUCOFED CH.32 + see PSEUDOEPHEDRINE, CODEINE
NUMORPHAN CH.51 OXYMORPHONE
NUPRIN CH.53 IBUPROFEN
NYLIDRIN CH.67 ARLIDIN
NYSTATIN CH.42 MYCOSTATIN
NYSTATIN CH.42 NILSTAT

O

OCTAMIDE CH.48 METOCLOPRAMIDE
OFLOXACIN CH.41 FLOXIN
OGEN CH.40 ESTROPIPATE
OMEPRAZOLE CH.20 PRILOSEC
OMNIPEN CH.55 AMPICILLIN
ONCOVIN CH.52 VINCRISTINE
OPTILET-500 CH.79 MULTIVITAMIN
OPTILET-M500 CH.79 MULTIVITAMIN
OPTIMINE CH.17 AZATADINE

P

PAPAVERINE CH.67 GENABID
PAPAVERINE CH.67 PAVABID
PARAFLEX CH.50 CHLORZOXAZONE
PARAFON FORTE DSC CH.50 CHLORZOXAZONE
PARAMETHASONE CH.60 HALDRONE
PARAPLATIN CH.5 CARBOPLATIN
PAREGORIC CH.51 TINC OPIUM CAMPHORATED
PAREGORIC CH.51 PG
PARGYLINE CH.46 EUTONYL
PARGYLINE, METHYCLOTHIAZIDE CH.46 EUTRON
PARNATE CH.46 TRANYLCYPROMINE
PATHILON CH.12 TRIHEXETHYL
PATHOCIL CH.55 HETACILLIN
PAVABID CH.67 PAPAVERINE
PAXIPAM CH.11 HALAZEPAM
PBZ CH.17 TRIPELENNAMINE
PBZ-SR CH.17 TRIPELENNAMINE
PCE CH.39 ERYTHROMYCIN
PEDIACOF CH.31 + see CPM, PHENYLEPHRINE, COD, POTASSIUM IODIDE
PEDIAPRED CH.60 PREDNISOLONE
PEDIAPROFEN CH.53 IBUPROFEN
PEDIAZOLE CH.61 + see ERYTHROMYCIN, SULFISOXAZOLE
PEGANONE CH.14 ETHOTOIN
PEMOLINE CH.30 CYLERT
PEN-G CH.55 PENICILLIN G
PEN-VEE-K CH.55 PENICILLIN V
PENBUTALOL CH.24 LEVATOL
PENICILLIN CH.55 ROBICILLIN V
PENICILLIN CH.55
PENICILLIN G CH.55 PEN-G
PENICILLIN G CH.55 PENTIDS
PENICILLIN V CH.55 BEEPEN-VK
PENICILLIN V CH.55 BETAPEN-VK
PENICILLIN V CH.55 LEDERCILLIN
PENICILLIN V CH.55 PEN-VEE-K
PENICILLIN V CH.55 PENICILLIN VK
PENICILLIN V CH.55 V-CILLIN-K
PENICILLIN V CH.55 VEETIDS
PENICILLIN VK CH.55 PENICILLIN V
PENNTUSS CH.32 + see CHLORPHENIRAMINE, CODEINE
PENTAERYTHRITOL TETRANITRATE CH.67 PERITRATE

PHENERGAN-D CH.18 PROMETNAZINE, PSEUDOEPHDRINE
PHENINDAMINE CH.17 NOLAHIST
PHENIRAMINE, PPA, PYRILAMINE, P-TOLOXAMINE CH.18 POLY-HISTINE-D
PHENIRAMINE, PYRILAMINE, PPA, HYDROCODONE, GG CH.32 TRIAMINIC-DH
PHENIRAMINE, PYRILAMINE, TERPIN HYDRATE, APAP CH.31 TUSSAGESIC
PHENOBARBITAL CH.23 LUMINAL
PHENSUXIMIDE CH.15 MILONTIN
PHENTERMINE CH.30 ADIPEX-P
PHENTERMINE CH.30 FASTIN
PHENTERMINE CH.30 IONAMIN
PHENYLBUTAZONE CH.53 BUTAZOLIDIN
PHENYLBUTAZONE CH.53 PHENYLBUTAZONE
PHENYLEPHRINE, DEXTROMETHORPHAN CH.32 CONAR
PHENYLEPHRINE, DEXTROMETHORPHAN, GUIAFENESIN CH.32 CONAR EXP
PHENYLEPHRINE, DEXTROMETHORPHAN, GUAIFENESIN, APAP CH.32 CONAR-A
PHENYLPROPANOLAMINE CH.33 ACUTRIM
PHENYLPROPANOLAMINE CH.33 DEXATRIM
PHENYLPROPANOLAMINE CH.33 PPA
PHENYLPROPANOLAMINE CH.33 PROPADRINE
PHENYLPROPANOLAMINE CH.33 PROPAGEST
PHENYLPROPANOLAMINE, HYDROCODONE CH.32 CODAMINE
PHENYLPROPANOLAMINE, HYDROCODONE CH.32 HYCOMINE
PHENYLPROPANOLAMINE, CODEINE, GUAIFENESIN CH.32 NALDECON-CX
PHENYLPROPANOLAMINE, DM, GUAIFENESIN CH.32 ROBITUSSIN CF
PHENYLPROPANOLAMINE, CARAMIPHEN CH.32 TUSS-GENADE
PHENYLPROPANOLAMINE, CARAMIPHEN CH.32 TUSS-ORNADE
PHENYLPROPANOLOAMINE, GUAIFENESIN CH.31 POLYHISTINE-Ex
PHENYLTOLOXAMINE, PPA, ACETAMINOPHEN CH.18 SINUBID
PHENYTOIN CH.14 DILANTIN
PHENYTOIN, PHENOBARBITAL CH.14 DILANTIN-PB
PHRENILIN CH.23 + see BUTALBITAL, ACETAMINOPHEN
PHYTONADIONE CH.78 MEPHYTON
PINDOLOL CH.24 VISKEN

INDEX

POTASSIUM CHLORIDE CH.57 KLOTRIX
POTASSIUM CHLORIDE, POTASSIUM GLUCONATE CH.57 KOLYUM
POTASSIUM CHLORIDE CH.57 MICRO-K
POTASSIUM CHLORIDE CH.57 RUM-K SF
POTASSIUM CITRATE, POTASSIUM GLUCONATE CH.57 TWIN-K
POTASSIUM GLUCONATE CH.57 KAON
POTASSIUM IODIDE SAT. SOL. CH.31 SSKI
POTASSIUM PHOSPHATES CH.57 K-PHOS
POTASSIUM PRODUCTS CH.57
PPA CH.33 PHENYLPROPANOLAMINE
PRAMET-FA CH.77+79 VITAMINS, FOLIC ACID
PRAMILET-FA CH.77+79 VITAMINS, FOLIC ACID
PRAVACHOL CH.29 PRAVASTATIN
PRAVASTATIN CH.29 PRAVACHOL
PRAZEPAM CH.11 CENTRAX
PRAZOSIN CH.6 MINIPRESS
PRAZOSIN, POLYTHIAZIDE CH.6 MINIZIDE
PREDNISOLONE CH.60 PEDIAPRED
PREDNISONE CH.60 DELTASONE
PREDNISONE CH.60 LIQUID PRED
PREDNISONE CH.60 METICORTEN
PREDNISONE CH.60 ORASONE
PRELU-2 CH.30 PHENDIMETRAZINE
PRELUDIN CH.30 PHENDIMETRAZINE
PREMARIN CH.40 ESTROGENS CONJUGATED
PRENATAL-S CH.79 MULTIVITAMIN
PRILOSEC CH.20 OMEPRAZOLE
PRIMIDONE CH.15 MYSOLINE
PRINCIPEN CH.55 AMPICILLIN
PRINIVIL CH.2 LISINOPRIL
PRINZIDE CH.2 + see LISINOPRIL, HYDROCHLOROTHIAZIDE
PRO-BANTHINE CH.12 PROPANTHELINE
PROBEC-T CH.79 MULTIVITAMIN
PROBEN/COLCH CH.43 + see PROBENECID, COLCHICINE
PROBENECID CH.43 BENEMID
PROBENECID, COLCHICINE CH. 43 COLBENEMID
PROBENECID, COLCHICINE CH. 43 PROBEN/COLCH
PROBUCOL CH.29 LORELCO
PROCAINAMIDE CH.21 PROCAN SR
PROCAINAMIDE CH.21 PRONESTYL
PROCAINAMIDE CH.21 PRONESTYL SR

PROTIPTYLINE CH.16 VIVACTIL
PROTOSTAT CH.49 METRONIDAZOLE
PROVENTIL CH.25 ALBUTEROL
PROVERA CH.40 MEDROXYPROGESTERONE
PROZAC CH.16 FLUOXETINE
PSEUDOEPHEDRINE CH.33 AFRINOL
PSEUDOEPHEDRINE CH.33 NOVAFED
PSEUDOEPHEDRINE CH.33 SUDAFED
PSEUDOEPHEDRINE, CHLORPHENIRAMINE CH.18 SUDAFED PLUS
PSEUDOEPHEDRINE, CODEINE, GUIAFENESIN CH.32 NOVAHISTINE EXP
PSEUDOEPHEDRINE, CODEINE CH.32 NUCOFED
PSEUDOEPHEDRINE, CODEINE CH.32 NUCOFED
PSEUDOEPHEDRINE, DEXTROMETHORPHAN, GG CH.32 RU-TUSS EXP
PSEUDOEPHEDRINE, CODEINE, GUAIFENESIN CH.32 RYNA-CX
PURINETHOL CH.5 MERCAPTOPURINE
PYRIDOXINE CH.72 HEXA-BETALIN
PYRIDOXINE CH.72 VITABEE 6
PYRIDOXINE CH.72 VITAMIN B-6
PYRILAMINE, PHENYLEPHRINE, DEXTROMETHORPHAN CH.32 CODIMAL DM
PYRILAMINE, PHENYLEPHRINE, HYDROCODONE CH.32 CODIMAL-DH
PYRILAMINE, PHENYLEPHRINE, CODEINE CH.32 CODIMAL-PH
PYRROXATE CH.18 CHLORPHENIRAMINE, PHENYLPROPANOLAMINE, APAP

Q

QUARZAN CH.12 CLINDINIUM
QUESTRAN CH.29 CHOLESTYRAMINE
QUIBRON CH.63 + see THEOPHYLLINE, GUAIFENESIN
QUINAGLUTE CH.21 QUINIDINE
QUINAPRIL CH.2 ACCUPRIL
QUINESTROL CH.40 ESTROVIS
QUINETHAZONE CH.37 HYDROMOX
QUINIDEX CH.21 QUINIDINE
QUINIDINE CH.21 CARDIOQUIN
QUINIDINE CH.21 CIN QUIN
QUINIDINE CH.21 DURAQUIN
QUINIDINE CH.21 QUINIDEX
QUINIDINE CH.21 QUINORA
QUINIDINE GLUCONATE CH.21 QUINAGLUTE

RESPBID CH.63 THEOPHYLLINE
RESTORIL CH.11 TEMAZEPAM
RETROVIR CH.68 ZIDOVUDINE
RHEUMATREX CH.47 METHOTREXATE
RIOPAN CH.10 MAGALDRATE
RITALIN CH.30 METHYLPHENIDATE
ROBAXIN CH.50 METHOCARBAMOL
ROBAXISAL CH.50 + see METHOCARBAMOL, ASPIRIN
ROBICILLIN V CH.55 PENICILLIN
ROBIMYCIN CH.39 ERYTHROMYCIN
ROBINUL CH.12 GLYCOPYRROLATE
ROBITET CH.62 TETRACYCLINE
ROBITUSSIN CH.31 GUAIFENESIN
ROBITUSSIN AC CH.32 + see GUAIFENESIN, CODEINE
ROBITUSSIN CF CH.32 + see PHENYLPROPANOLAMINE, DM, GUAIFENESIN
ROBITUSSIN DAC CH.32 + see GUAIFENESIN, DEXTROMETHORPAN, CODEINE
ROBITUSSIN DM CH.32 + see GUAIFENESIN, DEXTROMETHORPAN
ROBITUSSIN PE CH.31 + see GUAIFENESIN, PHENYLEPHRINE
ROCALTROL CH.75 CALCITRIOL
ROCEPHIN CH.28 CEFTRIAXONE
ROFERON A CH.44 INTERFERON ALPHA 2A
ROLAIDS SF CH.10 CALCIUM, MAGNESIUM
RONDEC CH.18 CARBINOXAMINE, PSEUDOEPHEDRINE
RONDEC-DM CH.32 + see CARBINOXAMINE, PSEUDOEPHEDRINE, DM
RONDOMYCIN CH.62 METHACYCLINE
ROXANOL CH.51 MORPHINE
ROXICET CH.51 + see OXYCODONE, ACETAMINOPHEN
RU-TUSS CH.18 CHLORPHENIRAMINE, PHENYLEPHRINE
RU-TUSS EXP CH.32 + see PSEUDOEPHEDRINE, DM, GUIAFENESIN
RUBEX CH.52 DOXORUBICIN
RUBRAMIN-PC CH.73 VITAMIN B-12
RUFEN CH.53 IBUPROFEN
RUM-K SF CH.57 POTASSIUM CHLORIDE
RYNA-C CH.32 + see CHLORPHENIRAMINE, PSEUDOEPHEDRINE, CODEINE
RYNA-CX CH.32 + see PSEUDOEPHEDRINE, CODEINE, GUAIFENESIN

SINGLET CH.18 CHLORPHENIRAMINE, PHENYLPROPANOLAMINE, APAP
SINUBID CH.18 PHENYLTOLOXAMINE, PHENYLPROPANOLAMINE, APAP
SINUTAB CH.18 CHLORPHENIRAMINE, PSEUDOEPHEDRINE, ACETAMINOPHEN
SKELAXIN CH.50 METAXALONE
SLO-BID CH.63 THEOPHYLLINE
SLO-PHYLLIN CH.63 THEOPHYLLINE
SMZ-TMP CH.61 SULFAMETHOXAZOLE, TRIMETHOPRIM
SODIUM SALICYLATE CH.58 PABALATE
SOFARIN CH.13 WARFARIN
SOMA CH.50 CARISOPRODOL
SOMINEX FORM 2 CH.17 DIPHENHYDRAMINE
SOMOPHYLLIN CH.63 THEOPHYLLINE
SORBITRATE CH.67 ISOSORBIDE
SPARINE CH.65 PROMAZINE
SPECTROBID CH.55 BACAMPICILLIN
SPIRONO/HCTZ CH.36 + see SPIRONOLACTONE, HYDROCHLOROTHIAZIDE
SPIRONOLACTONE CH.36 ALDACTONE
SPIRONOLACTONE, HYDROCHLOROTHIAZIDE CH.36 ALDACTAZIDE
SPIRONOLACTONE, HYDROCHLOROTHIAZIDE CH.36 SPIRONO/HCTZ
SPIRONOLACTONE, HYDROCHLOROTHIAZIDE CH.36 SPIROZIDE
SPIROZIDE CH.36 + see SPIRONOLACTONE, HYDROCHLOROTHIAZIDE
SSKI CH.31 POTASSIUM IODIDE SAT. SOL.
STANOZOLOL CH.9 WINSTROL
STELAZINE CH.65 TRIFLUPERAZINE
STEROIDS CH.60
STREPTOZOCIN CH.5 ZANOSAR
STRESSTABS CH.79 MULTIVITAMIN
STUART PRENAT CH.79 MULTIVITAMIN
STUARTINIC CH.79 + see FERROUS SULFATE, VITAMINS
STUARTNATAL1+1 CH.79 MULTIVITAMIN
SUCRALFATE CH.20 CARAFATE
SUDAFED CH.33 PSEUDOEPHEDRINE
SUDAFED PLUS CH.18 PSEUDOEPHEDRINE, CHLORPHENIRAMINE

TAZICEF CH.28 CEFTAZIDIME
TEDRAL CH.63 + see THEOPHYLLINE, EPHEDRINE, PB
TEGOPEN CH.55 CLOXACILLIN
TEGRETOL CH.15 CARBAMAZEPINE
TEMARIL CH.17 TRIMEPRAZINE
TEMAZEPAM CH.11 RESTORIL
TEMPRA CH.3 ACETAMINOPHEN
TENEX CH.7 GUANFACINE
TENORETIC CH.24 + see ATENOLOL, CHLORTHALIDONE
TENORMIN CH.24 ATENOLOL
TENUATE CH.30 DIETHYLPROPION
TEPANIL CH.30 DIETHYLPROPION
TERAZOCIN CH.6 HYTRIN
TERBUTALINE CH.25 BRETHAIRE
TERBUTALINE CH.25 BRETHINE
TERBUTALINE CH.25 BRICANYL
TERFENADINE CH.17 SELDANE
TERFENADINE, PSEUDOEPHEDRINE CH.18 SELDANE-D
TERPIN HYDRATE, CODEINE CH.32 TH & C
TERRAMYCIN CH.62 OXYTETRACYCLINE
TESLAC CH.52 TESTOLACTONE
TESPA CH.5 THIOTEPA
TESSALON CH.32 BENZONATATE
TESTOLACTONE CH.52 TESLAC
TESTRED CH.9 METHYLTESTOSTERONE
TETRACYCLINE CH.62 ACHROMYCIN-V
TETRACYCLINE CH.62 PANMYCIN
TETRACYCLINE CH.62 ROBITET
TETRACYCLINE CH.62 SUMYCIN
TETRACYCLINES CH.62
TG CH.5 THIOGUANINE
TH & C CH.32 + see TERPIN HYDRATE, CODEINE
THALITONE CH.37 CHLORTHALIDONE
THEO-24 CH.63 THEOPHYLLINE
THEO-DUR CH.63 THEOPHYLLINE
THEOBID CH.63 THEOPHYLLINE
THEOCLEAR-LA CH.63 THEOPHYLLINE
THEOLAIR CH.63 THEOPHYLLINE
THEON CH.63 THEOPHYLLINE
THEOPHYLLINE CH.63 ACCURBRON
THEOPHYLLINE CH.63 BRONKODYL
THEOPHYLLINE CH.63 CONSTANT-T

THYROLAR CH.64 LIOTRIX
TIMOLIDE CH.24 + see TIMOLOL, HYDRCHLOROTHIAZIDE
TIMOLOL, HYDRCHLOROTHIAZIDE CH.24 TIMOLIDE
TINC OPIUM CAMPHORATED CH.51 PAREGORIC
TITRALAC CH.10 CALCIUM CARBONATE
TOCAINIDE CH.22 TONOCARD
TOFRANIL CH.16 IMIPRAMINE
TOLAZAMIDE CH.34 TOLINASE
TOLBUTAMIDE CH.34 ORINASE
TOLECTIN CH.53 TOLMETIN
TOLECTIN-DS CH.53 TOLMETIN
TOLINASE CH.34 TOLAZAMIDE
TOLMETIN CH.53 TOLECTIN
TOLMETIN-DS CH.53 TOLECTIN-DS
TONOCARD CH.22 TOCAINIDE
TOPROL XL CH.24 METOPROLOL
TORADOL CH.53 KETOROLAC
TORNALATE CH.25 BITOLTEROL
TOTACILLIN CH.55 AMPICILLIN
TRAL CH.12 HEXOCYCLIUM
TRANDATE CH.24 LABETALOL
TRANDATE HCT CH.24 + see LABETALOL, HCTZ
TRANQUILIZERS CH.65
TRANXENE CH.11 CLORAZEPATE
TRANYLCYPROMINE CH.46 PARNATE
TRAZODONE CH.16 DESYREL
TRI-HYDROSERPINE CH.4 + see RESERPINE, HYDRALAZINE, HCTZ
TRI-LEVLIN CH.54 LEVONORGESTREL, ETHINYL ESTRADIOL
TRI-NORINYL CH.54 NORETHINDRONE, ETHINYL ESTRADIOL
TRI-PHEN-CHLOR CH.18 CHLORPHENIRAMINE, PPA, PHENYLEPHRINE, P-TOLOX.
TRI-VI-FLOR CH.79 + see VITAMINS, FLUORIDE
TRIAMCINOLONE CH.60 ARISTO-PAK
TRIAMCINOLONE CH.60 ARISTOCORT
TRIAMCINOLONE CH.60 AZMACORT
TRIAMCINOLONE CH.60 KENACORT
TRIAMCINOLONE CH.60 KENALOG
TRIAMCINOLONE CH.60 NASACORT
TRIAMINIC CH.18 CHLORPHENIRAMINE, PHENYPROPANOLAMINE
TRIAMINIC-DH CH.32 + see PHENIRAMINE, PYRILAMINE, PPA, HYDROCODONE, GG

TUSQUELIN CH.32 + see CHLORPHENIRAMINE, PHENYLEPHRINE, PPA, DM
TUSS-GENADE CH.32 + see PHENYLPROPANOLAMINE, CARAMIPHEN
TUSS-ORNADE CH.32 + see PHENYLPROPANOLAMINE, CARAMIPHEN
TUSSAGESIC CH.31 + see PHENIRAMINE, PYRILAMINE, TERPIN HYDRATE, APAP
TUSSAR-2 CH.32 + see CHLORPHENIRAMINE, CODEINE, GG
TUSSAR-DM CH.32 + see CHLORPHENIRAMINE, PSEUDOEPHEDRINE, DM
TUSSAR-SF CH.32 + see CHLORPHENIRAMINE, CODEINE, GG
TUSSI-ORGANIDIN CH.31 + see CODIENE, IODINATED GLYCEROL
TUSSIONEX CH.32 + see HYDROCODONE, PHENYLTOLOXAMINE RESIN CO
TWIN-K CH.57 + see POTASSIUM CITRATE, POTASSIUM GLUCONATE
TY-TABS CH.3 ACETAMINOPHEN
TYLENOL CH.3 ACETAMINOPHEN
TYLENOL #2,3,4 CH.51 + see ACETAMINOPHEN, CODEINE
TYLENOL+COD CH.51 + see ACETAMINOPHEN, CODEINE
TYLOX CH.51 + see OXYCODONE, ACETAMINOPHEN

U

ULTRACEF CH.28 CEFADROXIL
UNIPEN CH.55 NAFCILLIN
UNIPHYL CH.63 THEOPHYLLINE
UNISOM CH.17 DOXYLAMINE
URACIL CH.5 URACIL MUSTARD
URACIL MUSTARD CH.5 URACIL
UREX CH.66 METHENAMINE HIPPURATE
URINARY ANTISEPTICS CH.66
URISED CH.66 + see METHENAMINE, ATROPINE, HYOSCYAMINE+
URITIN CH.66 + see METHENAMINE, ATROPINE, HYOSCYAMINE+
UROFOLLITROPIN CH.40 METRODIN
UROPLUS CH.61 + see SULFAMETHOXAZOLE, TRIMETHOPRIM

V

V-CILLIN-K CH.55 PENICILLIN V
VALADOL CH.3 ACETAMINOPHEN
VALIUM CH.11 DIAZEPAM
VALMID CH.59 ETHINAMATE
VALPIN-50 CH.12 ANISOTROPINE

INDEX